BROKEN
be made whole

A GUIDE TO YOUR HEALING

BY MARILYN HICKEY

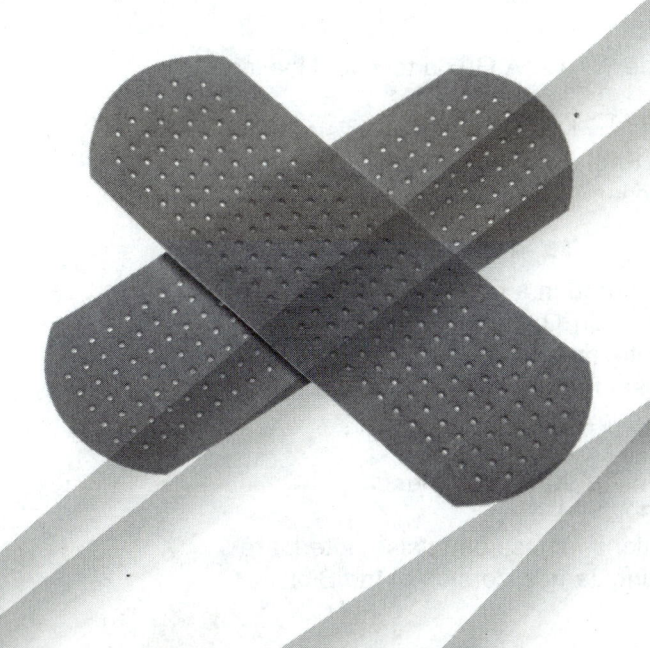

Broken, Be Made Whole: A Guide to Your Healing

Copyright © 2011 by Marilyn Hickey Ministries
P.O. Box 6598, Englewood, CO 80155
www.marilynandsarah.org

All rights reserved. No part of this publication may be reproduced, stored in a retrieval system or transmitted in any form by any means, electronic, mechanical, photocopy, recording or otherwise, without permission from publisher, except as provided by US copyright law.

Printed in the United States of America
ISBN 978-0-9830274-1-6
Scripture quotations, unless otherwise noted, are from the New King James Version of the Bible

TABLE OF CONTENTS

Section I – Receive Your Healing

Chapter One	Types of Healing
Chapter Two	Faith Really Does Work!
Chapter Three	The Prayer of Faith
Chapter Four	Faith and Confession
Chapter Five	Building Up Our Faith: Speak His Words

Section II – Keep Your Healing

Chapter Six	Don't Let Go
Chapter Seven	How Can I Keep Something I Haven't Received?
Chapter Eight	The Threat of a Storm
Chapter Nine	Fight the Good Fight

Section III – Sickness and Demons

Chapter Ten	Sickness
Chapter Eleven	Demons

Section IV – Healing the Sick

Chapter Twelve	The Power of Community
Chapter Thirteen	Methods God Uses

Appendices

INTRODUCTION

And [God] said, "If you diligently heed the voice of the LORD your God and do what is right in His sight, give ear to His commandments and keep all His statutes, I will put none of the diseases on you which I have brought on the Egyptians. For I am the LORD who heals you" (Exodus 15:26, NKJV).

I can't tell you how excited I am about this particular study, *Broken, Be Made Whole*. Fighting for good health is a hot topic of our day. Much of our time and money is spent on pursuing health and healing. Medicine itself has become so specialized that we need a different doctor for every problem or body part. Large hospitals and medical centers etch the skyline of every major city and even the smallest of towns boast of a clinic. Trillions of dollars are spent on finding cures and the cost to stay well is staggering. And we also have more natural options than ever before in preventative medicine. Nutrition stores, herbs, natural remedies—all these things are a part of our lives, and yet we know we still have sick people everywhere.

There are many different reasons why we find ourselves sick. Some diseases are hereditary; some are from lack of proper nutrition; and other illnesses aren't even fully understood by doctors and there are no known cures. I appreciate what medical science is doing to improve our health, and I am thankful for every doctor practicing his skills to provide healing for our bodies. However, we know there are things they cannot do. In our sicknesses, we find ourselves in helpless situations in need of God's comfort and relief.

Known as the Great Physician, Jesus came to heal us, but I believe the church needs to be reminded of all that Scripture teaches about how He really wants to make us well—in body, soul, and spirit. This process involves community and the prayers of others. We all need to come alongside one another and pray for the broken and the sick, so we can be whole and live at our full potential.

This syllabus is a written workshop of how to pray for your healing and the healing of others. There are stigmas within our culture that the gift of healing is attached to the power of a single personality and is something that God did not give freely to all of us, the ordinary Christians. We've forgotten the power of "Christ in us" and sometimes only acknowledge the power of Christ in a big platform or a well-known ministry or a seasoned Christian whom we think is more spiritual than ourselves. Maybe we have been turned off by those who go through the big hype and sensationalize the simple request of asking for healing. As a woman who has experienced restored health in body, soul, and spirit, throughout this study I want to encourage you and point you toward Jesus, the Healer.

With deep gratitude,

Marilyn

Marilyn

Before we move into our first chapter, I do want you to take a moment and think about specific people who you want to pray for throughout these chapters who are in pain, whether it is physical or emotional (see prayer journal, Appendix A).

REFLECTION QUESTIONS

1. What are some barriers that keep you from praying for healing, whether it is for you or for others?

_____
_____
_____
_____
_____
_____
_____

2. What questions do you have about praying for healing?

_____
_____
_____
_____
_____
_____
_____
_____
_____
_____
_____
_____
_____
_____
_____
_____
_____

section 1

RECEIVE YOUR HEALING

CHAPTER ONE
TYPES OF HEALING

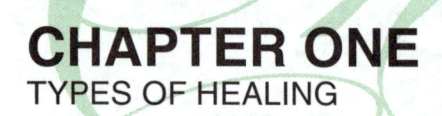

"And the very God of peace sanctify you wholly; and I pray God your whole spirit and soul and body be preserved blameless unto the coming of our Lord Jesus Christ" (1 Thessalonians 5:23, KJV).

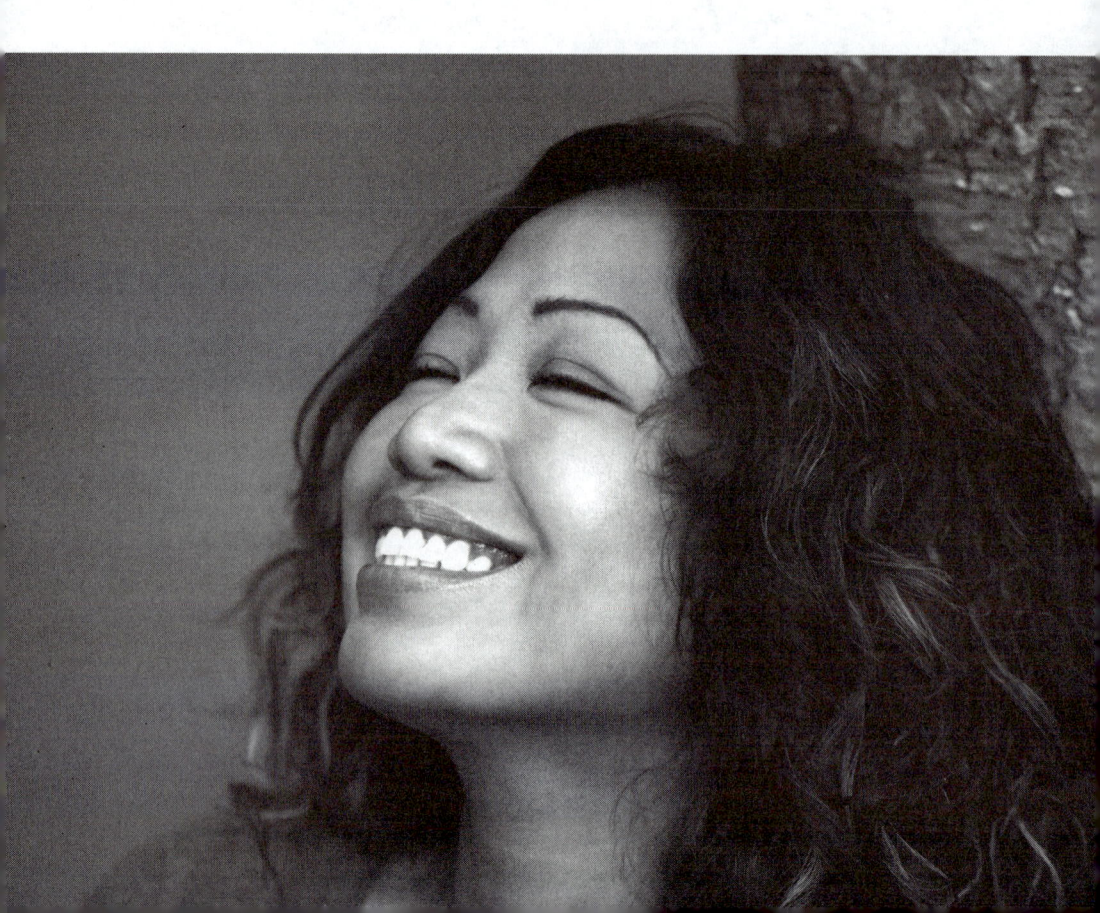

When we talk about healing, we usually are thinking of physical healing; but God's healing is for the whole person. Before we can understand the full gamut of healing we have to understand the different kinds humanity needs. Throughout Scripture, we see there are three types of healing in Jesus' ministry: body, soul, and spirit. His Word declares that healing is for our entire being.

THE SPIRIT

Paul put the spirit first. Without spirit wholeness, neither your soul nor your body can stay in good health—this must be a priority. Spirit wholeness means having the eternal life of God in your spirit by asking Jesus to be your Savior. Spirit "wellness" is maintained by following Him in every area of your life and submitting to the truth in His Word.

You may be someone who has been a follower of Christ for years or you may be a new believer. It really doesn't matter—we all can pray for the salvation of others. The "spirit" refers to the immaterial facet of humanity. Scripture tells us we are spiritually alive through Christ (1 Corinthians 2:11; Hebrews 4:12; James 2:26); and those who have not received the gift of salvation are not whole (Ephesians 2:1-5; Colossians 2:13). Our spirit gives us the ability to have an intimate relationship with God, who is said to be Spirit in John 4:24.

WORDS OF HEALING
TEXT: John 3:1-21 (MSG)

Nicodemus and Jesus

[1-2] There was a man of the Pharisee sect, Nicodemus, a prominent leader among the Jews. Late one night he visited Jesus and said, "Rabbi, we all know you're a teacher straight from God. No one could do all the God-pointing, God-revealing acts you do if God weren't in on it."

[3] Jesus said, "You're absolutely right. Take it from me: Unless a person is born from above, it's not possible to see what I'm pointing to—to God's kingdom."

[4] "How can anyone," said Nicodemus, "be born who has already been born and grown up? You can't re-enter your mother's womb and be born again. What are you saying with this 'born-from-above' talk?"

[5-6] Jesus said, "You're not listening. Let me say it again. Unless a person submits to this original creation—the 'wind-hovering-over-the-water' creation, the invisible moving the visible, a baptism into a new life—it's not possible to enter God's kingdom. When you look at a baby, it's just that: a body you can look at and touch. But the person who takes shape within is formed by something you can't see and touch—the Spirit—and becomes a living spirit.

[7-8] "So don't be so surprised when I tell you that you have to be 'born from above'—out of this world, so to speak. You know well enough how the wind blows this way and that. You hear it rustling through the trees, but you have no idea where it comes from or where it's headed next. That's the way it is with everyone 'born from above' by the wind of God, the Spirit of God."

[9] Nicodemus asked, "What do you mean by this? How does this happen?"

[10-12] Jesus said, "You're a respected teacher of Israel and you don't know these

basics? Listen carefully. I'm speaking sober truth to you. I speak only of what I know by experience; I give witness only to what I have seen with my own eyes. There is nothing secondhand here, no hearsay. Yet instead of facing the evidence and accepting it, you procrastinate with questions. If I tell you things that are plain as the hand before your face and you don't believe me, what use is there in telling you of things you can't see, the things of God?

13-15 "No one has ever gone up into the presence of God except the One who came down from that Presence, the Son of Man. In the same way that Moses lifted the serpent in the desert so people could have something to see and then believe, it is necessary for the Son of Man to be lifted up—and everyone who looks up to him, trusting and expectant, will gain a real life, eternal life.

16-18 "This is how much God loved the world: He gave his Son, his one and only Son. And this is why: so that no one need be destroyed; by believing in him, anyone can have a whole and lasting life. God didn't go to all the trouble of sending his Son merely to point an accusing finger, telling the world how bad it was. He came to help, to put the world right again. Anyone who trusts in him is acquitted; anyone who refuses to trust him has long since been under the death sentence without knowing it. And why? Because of that person's failure to believe in the one-of-a-kind Son of God when introduced to him.

19-21 "This is the crisis we're in: God-light streamed into the world, but men and women everywhere ran for the darkness. They went for the darkness because they were not really interested in pleasing God. Everyone who makes a practice of doing evil, addicted to denial and illusion, hates God-light and won't come near it, fearing a painful exposure. But anyone working and living in truth and reality welcomes God-light so the work can be seen for the God-work it is."

Nicodemus was a Pharisee and thought to be a prominent leader within the Jewish culture. There was a lot at stake for him in approaching Jesus; he chose to come to him at night and Jesus opened up to Nicodemus with open arms. It appears here that Nicodemus received the truth and believed he needed to be born again and renewed by the Spirit. Nicodemus, though he had prestige and power, knew the truth—that he was not yet whole—and received the gift of salvation. For the first time, this religious leader knew that the kingdom of God was not based on works, but the work of the Spirit. He acknowledged his ignorance and believed the truths Jesus was speaking to him. As soon as Nicodemus had the opportunity to understand, he received Jesus' truth. He is mentioned in other places in John, one where he is defending Jesus before the Jewish leaders (John 7:45-51), and then later with Joseph of Arimathea where they were preparing Jesus' body for burial (John 19:39-42).

God created us as spiritual beings. If we do not worship God, we will worship something or someone. And we will not be complete without the gift of salvation. Ephesians 2:8-9 says: *"For it is by grace you have been saved, through faith—and this is not from yourselves, it is a gift of God—not by works, so that no one can boast."*

INSIGHTS ON HEALING

1. Why do you think it is so hard for us/others to accept Jesus' free gift of salvation?

2. What are some of the issues Nicodemus struggled with when he went to Jesus?

3. How has the gift of salvation healed your spirit in ways you can recognize? Write some of them down.

THE SOUL

God also is concerned about the health of our soul. The word "soul" can refer to both the immaterial and material aspects of humanity; it's made up of your mind, your emotions, and also your will. Soul actually means "life." The Bible speaks of the soul in many contexts. Our soul has been affected by the Fall and only God can restore what we have lost because of sin that is present in the world. The soul, as with the spirit, is the center of many spiritual and emotional experiences (Job 30:25; Psalm 43:5; Jeremiah 13:17). Often, it refers to the whole person. Our soul and our spirit are connected but they are also separate. The soul is who we are, our essence. In the life of Jesus' ministry we see many times He knows the condition of a soul and heals its sickness. He can heal us when we have a broken heart—He can even heal our attitudes.

Soul sickness can result when we choose to hold onto anger or bitterness. Sometimes it is a result of not forgiving others—or one's self. Guilt is a terrible tormentor. Our souls can be sick when we have chosen a sinful pattern though we know what God's truth says. We do have doctors and therapists who can help us heal our souls and often God uses these resources. Yet it is wonderful to know He also will heal our souls.

WORDS OF HEALING
TEXT: John 4:1-30 (MSG)

Jesus and the Samaritan Woman

₁₋₃Jesus realized that the Pharisees were keeping count of the baptisms that he and John performed (although his disciples, not Jesus, did the actual baptizing). They had posted the score that Jesus was ahead, turning him and John into rivals in the eyes of the people. So Jesus left the Judean countryside and went back to Galilee.

₄₋₆To get there, he had to pass through Samaria. He came into Sychar, a Samaritan village that bordered the field Jacob had given his son Joseph. Jacob's well was still there. Jesus, worn out by the trip, sat down at the well. It was noon.

₇₋₈A woman, a Samaritan, came to draw water. Jesus said, "Would you give me a drink of water?" (His disciples had gone to the village to buy food for lunch.)

₉The Samaritan woman, taken aback, asked, "How come you, a Jew, are asking me, a Samaritan woman, for a drink?" (Jews in those days wouldn't be caught dead talking to Samaritans.)

₁₀Jesus answered, "If you knew the generosity of God and who I am, you would be asking me for a drink, and I would give you fresh, living water."

₁₁₋₁₂The woman said, "Sir, you don't even have a bucket to draw with, and this well is deep. So how are you going to get this 'living water'? Are you a better man than our ancestor Jacob, who dug this well and drank from it, he and his sons and livestock, and passed it down to us?"

₁₃₋₁₄Jesus said, "Everyone who drinks this water will get thirsty again and again. Anyone who drinks the water I give will never thirst—not ever. The water I give will be an artesian spring within, gushing fountains of endless life."

₁₅The woman said, "Sir, give me this water so I won't ever get thirsty, won't ever have to come back to this well again!"

₁₆He said, "Go call your husband and then come back."

₁₇₋₁₈"I have no husband," she said.

"That's nicely put: 'I have no husband.' You've had five husbands, and the man you're living with now isn't even your husband. You spoke the truth there, sure enough."

₁₉₋₂₀"Oh, so you're a prophet! Well, tell me this: Our ancestors worshiped God at this mountain, but you Jews insist that Jerusalem is the only place for worship, right?"

₂₁₋₂₃"Believe me, woman, the time is coming when you Samaritans will worship the Father neither here at this mountain nor there in Jerusalem. You worship guessing in the dark; we Jews worship in the clear light of day. God's way of salvation is made available through the Jews. But the time is coming—it has, in fact, come—when what you're called will not matter and where you go to worship will not matter.

₂₃₋₂₄"It's who you are and the way you live that count before God. Your worship must engage your spirit in the pursuit of truth. That's the kind of people the Father is out looking for: those who are simply and honestly themselves before him in their worship. God is sheer being itself—Spirit. Those who worship him must do it out of their very being, their spirits, their true selves, in adoration."

₂₅The woman said, "I don't know about that. I do know that the Messiah is coming. When he arrives, we'll get the whole story."

₂₆"I am he," said Jesus. "You don't have to wait any longer or look any further."

₂₇Just then his disciples came back. They were shocked. They couldn't believe he was talking with that kind of a woman. No one said what they were all thinking, but their faces showed it.

₂₈₋₃₀The woman took the hint and left. In her confusion she left her water pot. Back in the village she told the people, "Come see a man who knew all about the things I did, who knows me inside and out. Do you think this could be the Messiah?" And they went out to see for themselves.

In John 4, Jesus clearly healed the Samaritan woman's soul. She was taken into a pattern of adultery and her soul was broken because of sin. He healed her broken heart. She realized Jesus knew her inside and out. Though sometimes we don't even know what is going on in our soul, God does.

INSIGHTS ON HEALING

Prayerfully read over the passage about the Samaritan woman two times.

1. What are some unique things about the Samaritan woman's healing?

2. How did Jesus' words bring about healing? What did He do for her?

3. Sometimes we are stuck in despair and don't realize the cause. Jesus, however, knows the cause of all despair. If you desire for God to heal you of a fear or from a broken heart, take time to pray with someone. If you are alone right now, let the Spirit speak to you about this. Write out what you sense the Spirit is telling you.

HEALING ENCOUNTER

"He reveals the deep things of darkness and brings deep shadows into the light" (Job 12:22, NIV).

I was very sick several years ago and found out I had contracted parasites from traveling overseas. I was discouraged because I felt sick. I struggled to be around people and wanted to be alone. The darkness overwhelmed me at times. Not realizing it, I allowed the enemy to enter into a place in my heart at some level. A man my family trusted came and prayed with me, and while he prayed the LORD spoke to me about when I was eleven years old and my uncle sexually abused me. Now, I had long forgotten about that, but in that prayer time God revealed to me there was a hold on my heart. When this happened as a child, I believed it was my fault and I wanted to commit suicide. God brought this to me and all this time, the incident was there with me. Though this was a very hurtful time, I still was a top student; I was valedictorian and continued to have great successes in school. But years later, I had no idea it was still bothering me and didn't understand the source of my depression. I was praising God for three days after that time of prayer. There is no question: **He heals the brokenhearted**.

Read Job 12:22

1. Think about your own soul right now. Do you think there are things that have broken your heart but you might be unaware of what they are?

_____
_____
_____
_____
_____
_____
_____
_____
_____
_____
_____
_____
_____
_____
_____
_____
_____
_____
_____

2. Now write down the name of someone in your life that God is bringing to mind who needs healing in their soul. Picture them as a whole person. Write down what that looks like and how their life would be different. Take a moment to pray for them.

_____
_____
_____
_____
_____
_____
_____
_____
_____

THE BODY

As I travel overseas to poverty-stricken nations, it is hard to see the masses in need of medical relief. Yet there is no insurance or doctors that they can go to. I've found whether I am in a Muslim, Buddhist, or Hindu nation, most everyone welcomes prayers of healing. I can't tell you how encouraging it has been to see people healed at our events. I've found God to be faithful to heal, whether saved or unsaved. Many times healing brings an unbeliever to Christ. It can serve as the bridge to the LORD.

Sometimes I think when we see people who have been sick a long time, we think well that's chronic or they're older. But Scripture gives us many examples of people who had diseases for many years, like the man at the pool of Bethesda who was sick 38 years. Jesus saw him and healed him. Also, there was a woman who Satan had bound for 18 years with a spirit of infirmity. So, it doesn't matter how long you've been sick; you still can be healed. It's important to not get hung up on how long or how bad you think it is. The power is in Jesus' name.

If you are not convinced that God is your healer, I believe the Scriptures in this study will change your thinking.

WORDS OF HEALING
TEXT: Genesis 17; Genesis 18; Romans 4 (NIV)

Abraham and Sarah:
Genesis 17:2-6, 19-22

₂"I will confirm my covenant between me and you and will greatly increase your numbers."

₃Abram fell facedown, and God said to him, ₄"As for me, this is my covenant with you: You will be the father of many nations. ₅No longer will you be called Abram; your name will be Abraham, for I have made you a father of many nations. ₆I will make you very fruitful; I will make nations of you, and kings will come from you. ...

₁₉Then God said, "Yes, but your wife Sarah will bear you a son, and you will call him Isaac. I will establish my covenant with him as an everlasting covenant for his descendants after him. ₂₀And as for Ishmael, I have heard you: I will surely bless him; I will make him fruitful and will greatly increase his numbers. He will be the father of twelve rulers, and I will make him into a great nation. ₂₁But my covenant I will establish with Isaac, whom Sarah will bear to you by this time next year." ₂₂When he had finished speaking with Abraham, God went up from him.

Genesis 18:14

"Is anything too hard for the LORD? I will return to you at the appointed time next year and Sarah will have a son."

Romans 4:19-21

₁₉Without weakening in his faith, he faced the fact that his body was as good as dead—since he was about a hundred years old—and that Sarah's womb was also dead. ₂₀Yet he did not waver through unbelief regarding the promise of God, but was strengthened in his faith and gave glory to God, ₂₁being fully persuaded that God had power to do what he had promised.

INSIGHTS ON HEALING

1. What was Abraham's first response to God's miraculous promise?

2. How did Paul describe Abraham's faith in Romans 4?

3. Think about an impossible situation that requires God to heal someone physically. What verses in our text can you use to strengthen your faith? How does Abraham and Sarah's story minister to you personally?

_____
_____
_____
_____
_____
_____
_____
_____
_____
_____
_____
_____
_____
_____
_____
_____
_____
_____
_____
_____
_____
_____
_____
_____
_____
_____

God answers husbands when they pray for their wives. If you are a husband, be faithful to pray for your wife's physical health. If you are a wife, ask your husband to pray for your health continually, even if you are well.

HEALING ENCOUNTER

My heart overflowed with wonder and amazement when I saw the tiny bundle the nurse was handing to me. I pulled back the blanket and looked into the face of the most beautiful baby girl. I cuddled our precious Sarah—she truly was a gift from God. For thirteen years we cried out to the LORD for a child, and now the answer to our prayers wiggled in my arms. The doctors said, "Marilyn, you cannot bear children." But a man of God prophesied over me that Wally and I would have a child. Now, we did adopt our wonderful son, Michael, and I had accepted that as the fulfillment of God's promise, but Wally believed for a child of our flesh. And he was right!

I have seen the LORD perform miracle after miracle for childless couples, little miracles with names. The first healings in the Bible involved the healing of barren wombs. God has consistently proved throughout the history of humanity that He can create life when it is impossible.

HEALING ACTION POINT

Make a point to pray for someone who is struggling to have a child. We know God is the Giver of Life. Perhaps it is even you who is praying for this miracle. Begin to faithfully pray for God's healing hand and record your prayers and thoughts in your prayer journal in Appendix A.

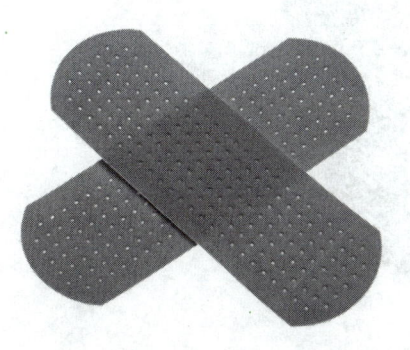

CHAPTER TWO
FAITH REALLY DOES WORK!

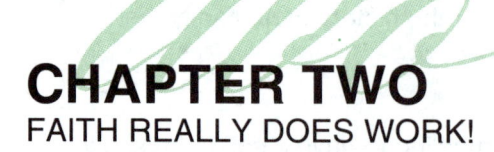

Now faith is the substance of things hoped for, the evidence of things not seen (Hebrews 11:1, NKJV).

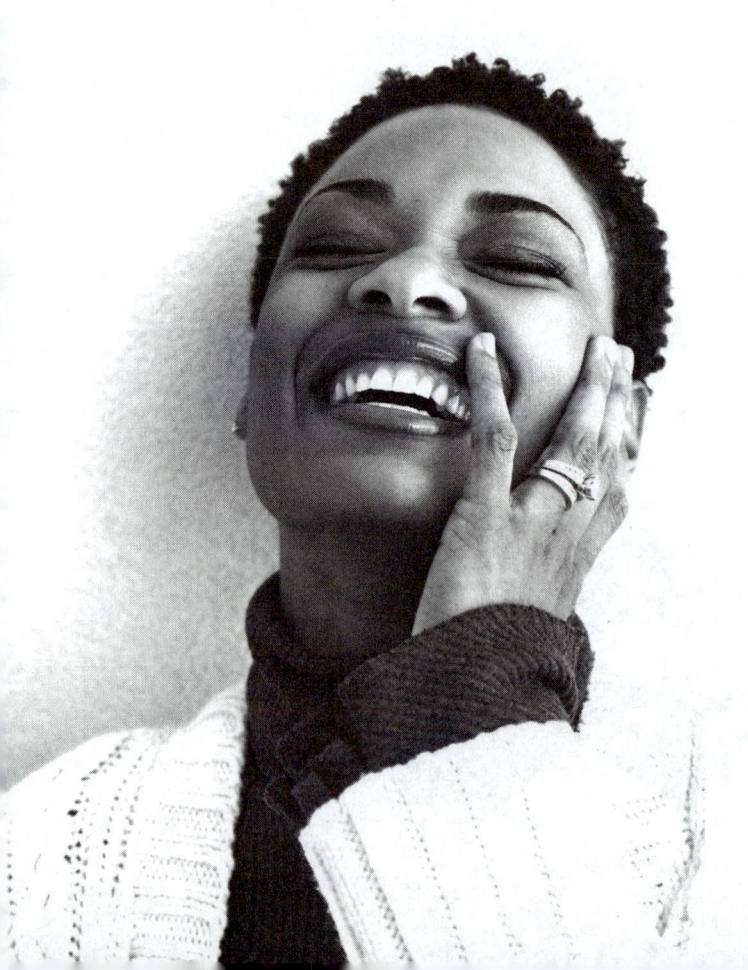

I want to share some simple thoughts about faith with you. I think the Word can trip us up and sometimes we make it more complicated than it is. You may read about Abraham being a man of faith and think, I can never have faith like Abraham. But really faith isn't measured by who we are; the focus should be on who God is. It isn't about us mustering up positive energy toward the universe or just positive thinking. Rather it is rooted in leaning into God and believing in Him.

Faith is: Believing God, today, is who He claims to be, that He can be trusted, and that His promises are true.

Faith is a now thing. God who dwells in eternity is a now God. God is eternal. He is not just future and past but all three. He is in a permanent state of being. Eternity is a spiritual realm. Faith gives us access to everything that exists in eternity. Faith brings it into the physical realm. Hebrews 11:1 says, "Now faith is the substance of things hoped for, the evidence of things not seen." Let's look closer at a few key words in this verse:

Substance is "hypostasis" which is a legal term of a title deed—the underlying reality. It is an established title deed. It is ownership when you have not seen it.

Evidence is "eleghos" which is certainty of something which we have yet to see. It is used in courts. Faith believes for invisible things.

The promises exist in eternity. The material realm is temporary. His Word is eternal. In the New Testament, the word faith is derived from the Greek word πίστις (pistis) or from the verb πιστεύω (pisteuo), meaning "to trust, to have confidence, faithfulness, to be reliable, to assure."

It's important to understand that the main source of faith is God Himself: First--Jesus, the Living Word; and Second--Scripture, the written Word. *While we do not look at the things which are seen, but at the things which are not seen. For the things which are seen are temporary, but the things which are not seen are eternal* (2 Corinthians 4:18, NKJV).

All things are created in the spiritual realm by God's Word.

As it is written, *"I have made you a father of many nations" in the presence of Him whom he believed—God, who gives life to the dead and calls those things which do not exist as though they did* (Romans 4:17, NKJV).

WORDS OF HEALING
Text: Mark 10:46-52 (NLT)

Jesus Heals a Blind Beggar
⁴⁶Then they reached Jericho, and as Jesus and his disciples left town, a large crowd followed him. A blind beggar named Bartimaeus (son of Timaeus) was sitting beside the road. ⁴⁷When Bartimaeus heard that Jesus of Nazareth was nearby, he

began to shout, "Jesus, Son of David, have mercy on me!"
⁴⁸"Be quiet!" many of the people yelled at him.
But he only shouted louder, "Son of David, have mercy on me!"
⁴⁹When Jesus heard him, he stopped and said, "Tell him to come here."
So they called the blind man. "Cheer up," they said. "Come on, he's calling you!"
⁵⁰Bartimaeus threw aside his coat, jumped up, and came to Jesus.
⁵¹"What do you want me to do for you?" Jesus asked.
"My rabbi," the blind man said, "I want to see!"
⁵²And Jesus said to him, "Go, for your faith has healed you." Instantly the man could see, and he followed Jesus down the road.

Throughout Scripture, we see many times when Jesus was moved by someone's faith in Him.

INSIGHTS ON HEALING

1. What was Bartimaeus' reaction when he learned that Jesus was nearby?

___

2. Why do you think Jesus asked Bartimaeus, "What do you want me to do for you?"

___

3. What are some barriers you feel are in the way of your healing, whether it is a physical sickness or, perhaps, an emotional one?

_____
_____
_____
_____
_____
_____
_____
_____
_____
_____
_____
_____

4. Reflect a moment if you have taken it before the LORD. Maybe you feel like you've pleaded and pleaded for His healing. Or maybe you know you have not asked or gone to Him enough. Explain, remembering He is present with you as you write out your thoughts.

_____
_____
_____
_____
_____
_____
_____
_____
_____
_____
_____
_____
_____

HEALING ENCOUNTER

Many of you know my heart for the lost and I love sharing about the healing power of Jesus. Traveling to so many different countries I have found a genuine openness to prayer, no matter if one is a Christian or Hindu. As I've shared with others about Jesus' healing it is amazing to me how eager He is to answer prayer.

Last spring I was invited to have a healing meeting in a mosque—that in itself was a miracle. In developing a relationship with the leaders of this mosque in Detroit, I was very clear with them. I said, "Yes, I would love to come and have a prayer meeting, but I pray in Jesus' name." Well, they were fine with that. Even in the Koran, there is reference to the fact that Jesus heals. I went and spoke and asked anyone to stand up who wanted prayer for a healing they needed. A few people stood up. Then I asked for testimonies, for anyone to share if they felt different. A young Muslim boy came forward and told me his eyes had been healed. There was a banner at the front of the mosque that he could not read before we prayed. He told me he could now read it perfectly. He believed that Jesus could heal him, even though his understanding of Jesus was limited. God's healing is for all people.

Healing is the bread of children—it's to be shared with others. Your faith in what Jesus can do can impact those around you. My team members who travel with me have been such a blessing. One time we were in Jakarta. We had a major meeting in a small stadium, perhaps five or six thousand people. My television crew was with me on this trip, and one was a nurse. She said to me, "I've prayed for healing for others but I've never had anyone come out of a wheelchair." So this was on her heart and she began praying ahead of time for a person in a wheelchair to come forward to her and that they would be healed. That night the whole team went up front so they could lay hands on the sick. A family came up to a woman on our travel team and said, "We've brought our father tonight. He's at the back in a wheelchair. She thought, "God, I'm scared. He's unconscious and in a wheelchair." You know it shook her. But then God spoke to her heart and said, "You know you've been believing I would send you this man." She made her way back to where the man was and laid hands on him and that man got out of the wheelchair. It was a dramatic miracle and we all celebrated in the faithfulness of God. Even when we have doubts that our prayers are even effective, our faith impacts others. We learn from each other and we need one another.

I like what theologian G.K. Chesterton says about miracles: "miracles ... they mean first, the freedom of the soul, and secondly, its control over the tyranny of circumstance."

"And the prayer of faith will save the sick, and the LORD will raise him up. And if he has committed sins, he will be forgiven" (James 5:15, NKJV).

HEALING ACTION POINT
Be open to what the Spirit speaks to you about what to pray for and who to pray for. Make sure you actively listen to the Spirit as you pray for others and make note of what He is saying to you in your prayer journal (Appendix A). Often He will lead you to the right Scriptures to pray over someone.

Notes:

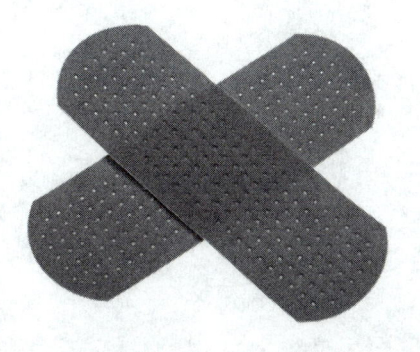

CHAPTER THREE

THE PRAYER OF FAITH

"And the prayer of faith will save the sick, and the LORD will raise him up. And if he has committed sins, he will be forgiven" (James 5:15, NKJV).

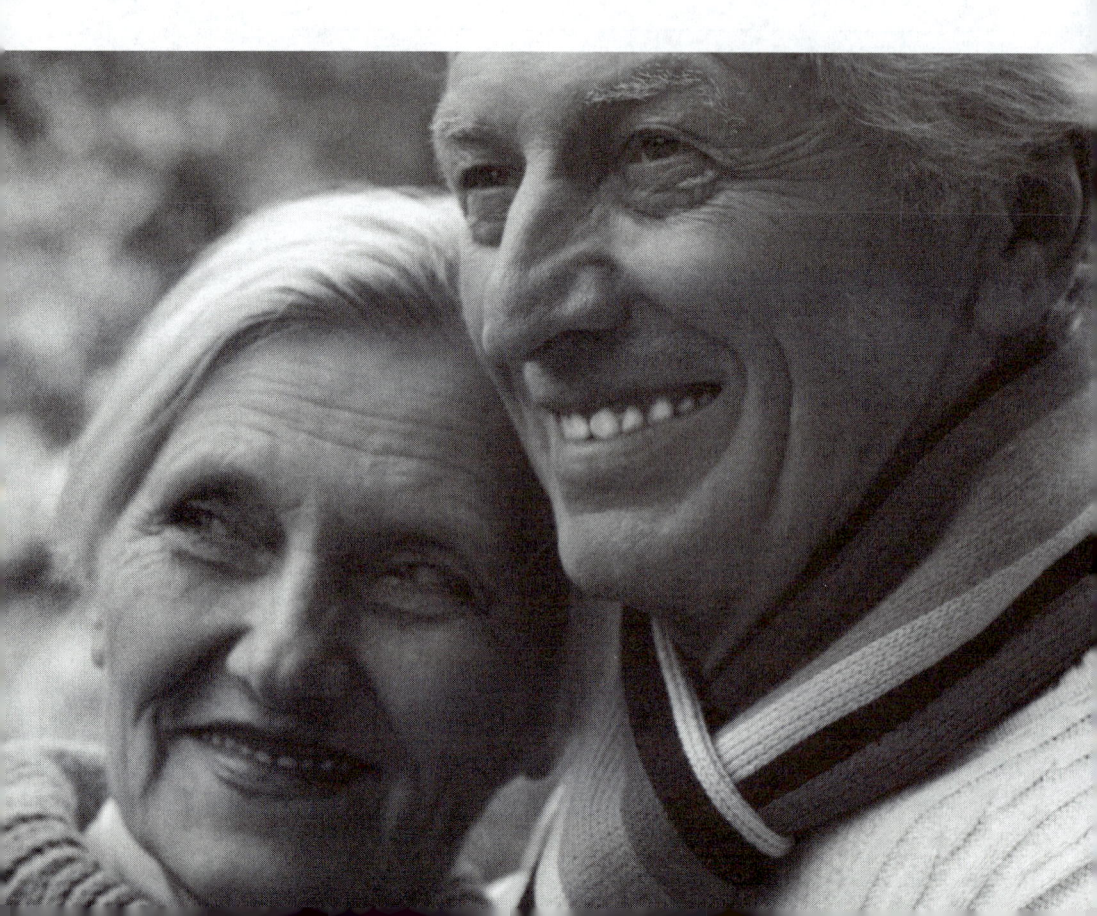

In the previous chapter we talked about what faith is and how simple it is to exercise it in your prayers for healing. You don't need the hype or high emotionalism to pray for someone and be effective. It is a matter of praying for your need, knowing God really is who He says He is: Jehovah Rapha, the God who heals.

And [God] said, "If you diligently heed the voice of the LORD your God and do what is right in His sight, give ear to His commandments and keep all His statutes, I will put none of the diseases on you which I have brought on the Egyptians. For I am the LORD who heals you" (Exodus 15:26, NKJV).

Through years of ministry I've found the enemy likes to deceive us by making us believe that God isn't going to answer a small prayer said by an ordinary person. Yet Scripture shows us that is not true. The disciples were extremely ordinary men; some were just fisherman looking to make a simple living. And yet God used their prayers and the sick were healed in Jesus' name. In Luke 10:17, the disciples came back and joyfully reported to him, "Lord, even the demons obey us when we use your name!" And Jesus told them, "Yes, I have given you authority over all the power of the enemy and you can walk among snakes and scorpions and crush them."

In the back of the syllabus is a prayer journal that I've mentioned in some of the Healing Action Points. My desire for you is to make efforts to pray for the sick around you and believe that your prayers can impact your friends, family, and even your enemies. Prayer is about community and is one of the best resources we have to connect to the eternal realm.

There are some church traditions that say that the gifts of the Spirit ceased after the last apostle. However, there is no Scripture to support that and the church is in the age of the Spirit—the gift Jesus left to His church. Or sometimes, we believe God heals people, but that miracles only happen overseas or on a mission field. Whatever perspective you have, I don't believe the church prays enough for the sick. At best, we mention those in the hospital in a newsletter or in our announcements but we don't seem convicted that our prayers of faith make a difference. Before we can offer up our prayers of faith, we have to believe they matter!

So you might say, "If I pray for the sick, how long do I need to pray? Is five minutes okay?" I will tell you from personal experience it doesn't take long at all. It's not how we feel or how long we pray, but rather that we actually do it. Starting with a better understanding of faith will help us to pray more willingly and more effectively.

Does faith have to be present for someone to be healed? This is a great question. In so many references in the Bible, God acknowledged the faith of the person being healed: Bartimaeus who was blind, the centurion who came to Jesus for his servant, the lame man at the Temple gate. I like to think of God's power as a stick of dynamite and faith as the fire that lights it.

But we know people get healed who have no faith in Christ or who are too weary to even try to pray. That's why the community of believers is important. Sometimes we need to invite others to lean on our faith. Or we should offer our prayers without them even knowing. Opportunities to pray for someone's healing can come when we are waiting in the check-out line at the grocery store. The enemy likes for us to think we could never have enough faith to be a catalyst toward someone's healing. The truth is we all get discouraged, especially if an answer doesn't come immediately. However, our faith can always be encouraged by others and renewed through the Word of God. The promises there are a never-ending source of supply.

WORDS OF HEALING
TEXT: Passages on Faith

"Blessed be the God and Father of our Lord Jesus Christ, who has blessed us with every spiritual blessing in the heavenly places in Christ" (Ephesians 1:3, NKJV).

"As His divine power has given to us all things that pertain to life and godliness, through the knowledge of Him who called us by glory and virtue, for by which have been given to us exceedingly great and precious promises, that through these you may be partakers of the divine nature, having escaped the corruption that is in the world through lust" (2 Peter 1: 3 – 4, NKJV).

"Who Himself bore our sins in His own body on the tree, that we, having died to sins, might live for righteousness — by whose stripes you were healed" (1 Peter 2:24, NKJV).

"For I say, through the grace given to me, to everyone who is among you, not to think of himself more highly than he ought to think, but to think soberly, as God has dealt to each one a measure of faith" (Romans 12:3, NKJV).

"So Jesus answered and said to them, "Have faith in God" (Mark 11:22, NKJV).

"I have been crucified with Christ; it is no longer I who live, but Christ lives in me; and the life which I now live in the flesh I live by faith in the Son of God, who loved me and gave Himself for me" (Galatians 2:20, NKJV).

"This only I want to learn from you: Did you receive the Spirit by the works of the law, or by the hearing of faith? Are you so foolish? Having begun in the Spirit, are you now being made perfect by the flesh? Have you suffered so many things in vain — if indeed it was in vain? Therefore He who supplies the Spirit to you and works miracles among you, does He do it by the works of the law, or by the hearing of faith?" (Galatians 3:2 – 5, NKJV).

INSIGHTS ON HEALING

1. Read over these passages carefully. Write your insights about what each passage is saying to you about faith: Ephesians 1:3; 2 Peter 1:3-4; 1 Peter 2:24; Romans 12:3; Mark 11:22; Galatians 2:20; Galatians 3:2-5.

2. What do you think Paul means when he says he now lives by faith?

3. What are some misconceptions you or others you know have had about faith?

HEALING ENCOUNTER

As you go through this study, you may develop a burden for people in your life who do not believe in healing and God may put opportunities right in front of you to share your faith with someone else.

A while back a friend asked me to come to her house and I didn't know why she was extending the invitation. She had serious arthritis and was leery about evangelists who believed in healing. "Marilyn, I don't like what I hear from some of these television evangelists, and I don't believe in healing. I have rheumatoid arthritis and I'm crippling up and can hardly do simple tasks anymore. You have faith, so you pray for me." And, so I did.

She now works full-time, sometimes ten, twelve-hour days with no arthritis. The doctor even told her that her blood had changed. My prayer was probably five minutes long and I didn't have a whole healing service to help her. You don't have to wait for a big meeting or for an evangelist to pray for a friend.

Start praying for someone who needs your faith!

HEALING ACTION POINT

It's helpful, too, if God has healed you from a sickness, to share that, then pray. For example, maybe you have had very painful arthritis. You could share this with a small group and then ask those with arthritis to stand because you want to pray for them. That wouldn't take long at all. Then ask those who stood to check for healing. Can you move a limb that you couldn't move before? Can anyone tell a difference? You may be using this syllabus as a Bible study. If so, take time in your group to practice praying for one another's healing. Begin sharing some testimonies of healing with one another.

It will take some courage to do this, but God will be faithful no matter what, whether or not anyone speaks up and shares a healing or not. In many cases, healing is a process, but that does not lessen the power of God at work.

Never limit what God can do. There is plenty of healing to go around.

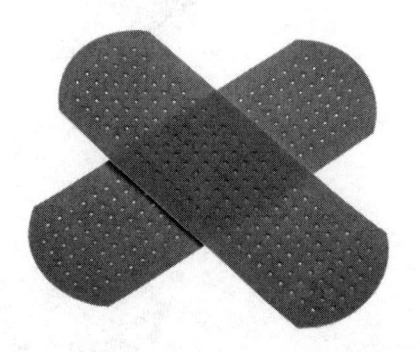

Notes:

CHAPTER FOUR

FAITH AND CONFESSION

"Then Jesus answered, 'Woman, you have great faith! Your request is granted.' And her daughter was healed from that very hour" (Matthew 15:28, NIV).

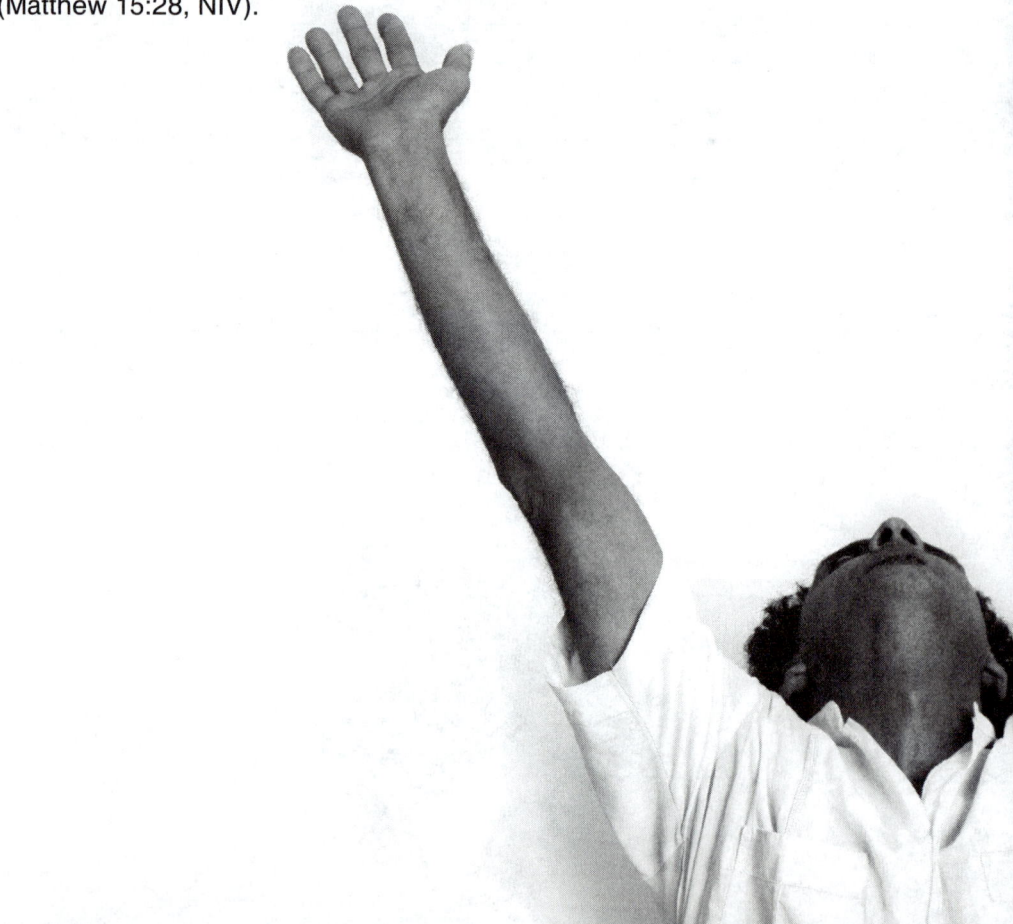

Our faith in God grows as we continue to get to know Him more, spend time in Scripture and learn about His promises. There are so many Scriptures that attest to His healing power. When we receive healing, it makes us want to worship Him. Something powerful happens when we worship God, and the enemy knows that, as he once was a beautiful worshiper in heaven.

There are three Greek words used for healing and in the New Testament Jesus' presence is involved. One is therapeuo, which means "to make whole." This word is used in Luke 5:1: One day, Jesus was standing by the Lake of Gennesaret with the people crowding around him and listening to the word of God. Here, the writer is emphasizing that the power of the LORD was present to heal. The Word is usually linked to worship and worship makes us whole. When we worship, we are aware of His unlimited power, we are moldable, and we are more open to His promises.

Haven't you found sometimes you can come into a worship service, be tired, depressed, and even sick but then you feel so much better after you worship God? Or maybe this has happened at home. You wake up in the night and things seem so bleak, so hopeless and you begin to worship. It's therapeutic and very healing. His presence heals us. Worship is something well beyond a church service. Keep yourself as much as possible in an atmosphere of worship, whether in the car, at work, or at home.

Another word for healing is sozo, which means "to restore to health." This can refer to when believers lay hands on the sick; some recover immediately and sometimes there is a process. This kind of healing can be for your spirit, your mind, or your body.

The third word is teleo, which means "to be complete." God completes His work; you are totally made well and whole. It relates to something accomplished, like when Jesus said from the cross, "It is finished." I'm a bit puzzled by Bible translators who sometimes do not include physical healing with His atoning work. Matthew 8:16-17 makes it clear that healing was in the atonement because it says:

"When evening came, many who were demon-possessed were brought to him, and he drove out the spirits with a word and healed all the sick. This was to fulfill what was spoken through the prophet Isaiah: "He took up our infirmities and carried our diseases (NIV).""

We are usually very open to the fact Jesus healed us spiritually but do not embrace that He also came to heal us physically.

"And if the Spirit of him who raised Jesus from the dead is living in you, he who raised Christ from the dead will also give life to your mortal bodies through his Spirit, who lives in you." (Romans 8:11, NIV)

As we begin to develop a heart for praying for the healing of others, it helps to understand that Jesus really did come to heal us—body, soul, and spirit. It's easy to gloss over all the Scriptures that attest this and become callous to these promises. A big part of cultivating prayers of faith comes from knowing what Scripture says.

WORDS OF HEALING
TEXT: Mark 7; Matthew 15 (NIV)

The Syrophenician Woman
Mark 7:25-30

25 In fact, as soon as she heard about him, a woman whose little daughter was possessed by an evil spirit came and fell at his feet. 26 The woman was a Greek, born in Syrian Phoenicia. She begged Jesus to drive the demon out of her daughter.
27 "First let the children eat all they want," he told her, "for it is not right to take the children's bread and toss it to their dogs."
28 "Yes, Lord," she replied, "but even the dogs under the table eat the children's crumbs."
29 Then he told her, "For such a reply, you may go; the demon has left your daughter."
30 She went home and found her child lying on the bed, and the demon gone.

Matthew 15:21-28

21 Leaving that place, Jesus withdrew to the region of Tyre and Sidon. 22 A Canaanite woman from that vicinity came to him, crying out, "Lord, Son of David, have mercy on me! My daughter is suffering terribly from demon-possession."
23 Jesus did not answer a word. So his disciples came to him and urged him, "Send her away, for she keeps crying out after us."
24 He answered, "I was sent only to the lost sheep of Israel."
25 The woman came and knelt before him. "Lord, help me!" she said.
26 He replied, "It is not right to take the children's bread and toss it to their dogs."
27 "Yes, Lord," she said, "but even the dogs eat the crumbs that fall from their masters' table."
28 Then Jesus answered, "Woman, you have great faith! Your request is granted." And her daughter was healed from that very hour.

This story is interesting for a few reasons. The woman was a Gentile, someone religious leaders would not think of as worthy of God's time. Sometimes we think only certain people deserve healing—but Jesus came to heal all people. The purpose of the story is to proclaim the healing abilities of Jesus and to explain the Jewish-Christian attitude toward the Gentiles. No believer at Corinth or Rome would find it necessary to question the validity of the exorcism's cure; Mark's readers are already convinced of Jesus' skills as a miracle worker: a Jewish rabbi hears the pleas of a Greek woman, effects a cure, and the cure is successful. And here, Jesus cures the daughter from a distance, not from a physical touch. The demon is exorcised by God's word alone—Jesus tells her the daughter has been healed.

INSIGHTS ON HEALING

1. Think of some prejudices you have toward those of another faith or lifestyle.

2. How does this account of healing challenge your theology or understanding about God?

3. What can we learn from the woman's faith?

HEALING ENCOUNTER

Clearly we see from Scripture that faith works. To illustrate, I witnessed a miracle in Little Rock, Arkansas several years ago. I felt led to pray for people with shoulder problems. I just invited people to stand and there were probably six or seven hundred people there that night. I don't know how many people stood up with shoulder problems, but the next night I asked for those to stand who wanted to share a testimony of healing.

Excitedly, a man stood up and shared, "I have a hole in my shoulder, right here in the bone. I can't lift my arm because of that hole. A burglar broke into my home and shot me. But this morning I didn't have on my pajama top while I was shaving and I looked at my shoulder and it looked like the hole was gone. Then I tried to lift my arm and realized God had healed me."

His gratitude was overflowing. Sometimes we think, well, faith just works for other people. But faith works in all settings, all countries, and through all of us.

HEALING ACTION POINT

Take time to go through the Gospels and underline a story of healing where Jesus says, "your faith has made you well" or he is amazed at someone's reply because they believed in Jesus' authority and confessed it.

"Faith is the confidence that what we hope for will actually happen; it gives us assurance about things we cannot see. Through their faith, the people in days of old earned a good reputation" (Hebrews 11:1-2, NLT).

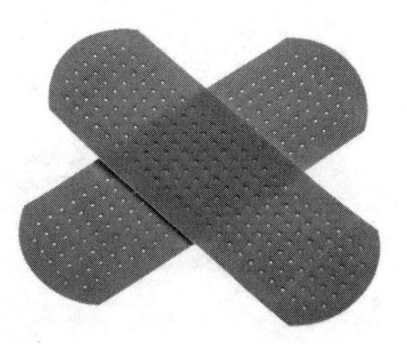

Notes:

CHAPTER FIVE

Building Up our Faith: Speak His Words

Health comes through His Word!—Marilyn

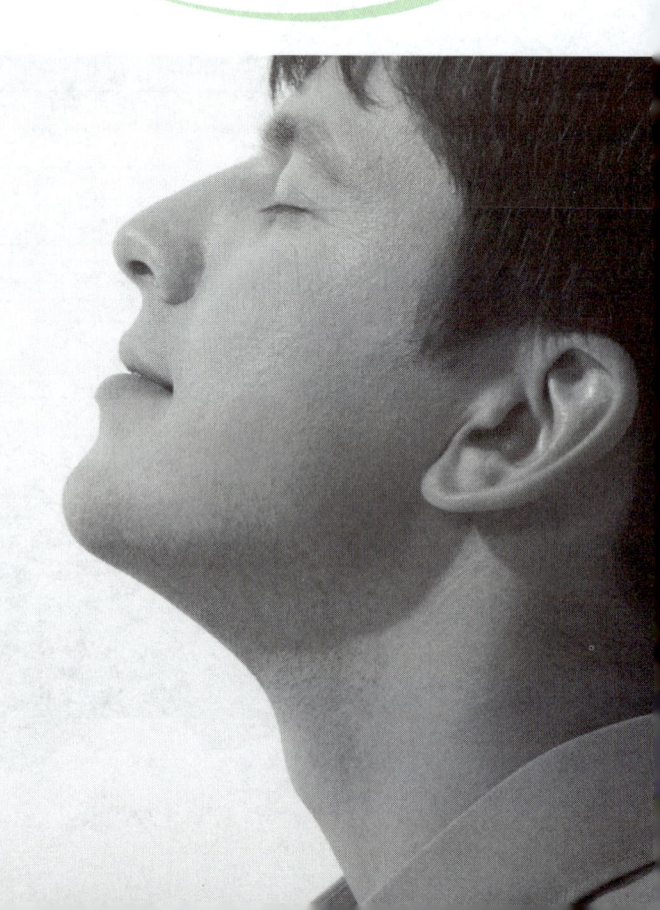

At this point in our study, we have read a lot of Scripture that affirms Jesus' desire to heal us. The more we read about His promises, the more our faith in Him will continue to grow, and the more we will speak His promises. We need to have confidence in His Word and begin to speak His Word to ourselves, in our prayers, and to others. Years ago, I put together a pamphlet, "Speak the Word" that encourages believers to meditate on His promises throughout the day.

Few things in life are as important as speaking God's Word everyday. When you confess His promises over your life and circumstances, your spouse and your children, things can change. Yet in our busy day-to-day lives, we often feel we just don't have the time. Here I want to share some key promises that you can begin to cultivate in your heart. Joshua 1:8 says:

"This book of the law shall not depart from your mouth, but you shall meditate on it day and night, so that you may be careful to do according to all that is written in it; for then you will make your way prosperous and then you will have success" (NASV).

Consider for a moment your thought life toward God and others. Do you confess more negative than positive things? When we hear ourselves speak God's Word our spirit hears it too. Our daily prayer should be, "Let the words of my mouth be acceptable in your sight today, O Lord."

There is so much bad news in the media that comes into our homes. It is hard to not feel the angst of all that is wrong with our communities and our nation. I'm not saying we should stick our head in the sand and dismiss the real global problems we have. God wants us to care about the world, and pray for it. The news changes daily, sometimes it is better the next day, sometimes not. But God's Word is constant and it is always true. Health comes through His Word. We need to renew our minds daily with His truth. 2 Corinthians 5:16-18 is a passage to memorize:

"That is why we never give up. For our present troubles are small and won't last very long. Yet they produce for us a glory that vastly outweighs them and will last forever! So we don't look at troubles we can see now; rather we fix our gaze on things that cannot be seen. For the things we see now will soon be gone, but the things we cannot see will last forever" (NLT).

God even goes as far to say that the unseen world is actually more real than the seen world which is temporal. The unseen world is eternal. God's point here is to not put our faith in things we can see, which will soon be gone. So we choose to put our faith in what we can't see and know God is at work.

I was at a wonderful church, a really strong church, praying for the sick. A Methodist man came to the meeting who had been in a car accident. He lost his eardrum, so he had no hearing in his left ear. He wasn't old, maybe in his 30s and he came forward for prayer and wanted to be saved. Well in the process of giving this to God, God gave him a new eardrum. He could hear perfectly out of his left ear. He went home and told his girlfriend what happened and she came to the next service and she also received Christ. People wanted to know Christ and we didn't have a baptismal but we brought in a tank so we could baptize them. Faith really does work. I didn't foresee the eardrum God gave him or how He was going to heal it. I just had faith in God. And faith is always a present-tense thing. God can do what He said He will do in all situations.

WORDS OF HEALING:
Text: Hebrews 11 (NIV)

By Faith
1Now faith is being sure of what we hope for and certain of what we do not see. 2This is what the ancients were commended for. 3By faith we understand that the universe was formed at God's command, so that what is seen was not made out of what was visible. 4By faith Abel offered God a better sacrifice than Cain did. By faith he was commended as a righteous man, when God spoke well of his offerings. And by faith he still speaks, even though he is dead.
5By faith Enoch was taken from this life, so that he did not experience death; he could not be found, because God had taken him away. For before he was taken, he was commended as one who pleased God. 6And without faith it is impossible to please God, because anyone who comes to him must believe that he exists and that he rewards those who earnestly seek him.
7By faith Noah, when warned about things not yet seen, in holy fear built an ark to save his family. By his faith he condemned the world and became heir of the righteousness that comes by faith.
8By faith Abraham, when called to go to a place he would later receive as his inheritance, obeyed and went, even though he did not know where he was going. 9By faith he made his home in the Promised Land like a stranger in a foreign country; he lived in tents, as did Isaac and Jacob, who were heirs with him of the same promise. 10For he was looking forward to the city with foundations, whose architect and builder is God.
11By faith Abraham, even though he was past age—and Sarah herself was barren—was enabled to become a father because he considered him faithful who had made the promise. 12And so from this one man, and he as good as dead, came descendants as numerous as the stars in the sky and as countless as the sand on the seashore.
13All these people were still living by faith when they died. They did not receive the things promised; they only saw them and welcomed them from a distance. And they admitted that they were aliens and strangers on earth. 14People who say such things show that they are looking for a country of their own. 15If they had been thinking of the country they had left, they would have had opportunity to return. 16Instead, they were longing for a better country—a heavenly one. Therefore God is not ashamed to be called their God, for he has prepared a city for them.
17By faith Abraham, when God tested him, offered Isaac as a sacrifice. He who had received the promises was about to sacrifice his one and only son, 18even though God had said to him, "It is through Isaac that your offspring will be reckoned." 19Abraham reasoned that God could raise the dead, and figuratively speaking, he

did receive Isaac back from death.

20By faith Isaac blessed Jacob and Esau in regard to their future.

21By faith Jacob, when he was dying, blessed each of Joseph's sons, and worshiped as he leaned on the top of his staff.

22By faith Joseph, when his end was near, spoke about the exodus of the Israelites from Egypt and gave instructions about his bones.

23By faith Moses' parents hid him for three months after he was born, because they saw he was no ordinary child, and they were not afraid of the king's edict.

24By faith Moses, when he had grown up, refused to be known as the son of Pharaoh's daughter. 25He chose to be mistreated along with the people of God rather than to enjoy the pleasures of sin for a short time. 26He regarded disgrace for the sake of Christ as of greater value than the treasures of Egypt, because he was looking ahead to his reward. 27By faith he left Egypt, not fearing the king's anger; he persevered because he saw him who is invisible. 28By faith he kept the Passover and the sprinkling of blood, so that the destroyer of the firstborn would not touch the firstborn of Israel.

29By faith the people passed through the Red Sea as on dry land; but when the Egyptians tried to do so, they were drowned.

30By faith the walls of Jericho fell, after the people had marched around them for seven days.

31By faith the prostitute Rahab, because she welcomed the spies, was not killed with those who were disobedient.

32And what more shall I say? I do not have time to tell about Gideon, Barak, Samson, Jephthah, David, Samuel and the prophets, 33who through faith conquered kingdoms, administered justice, and gained what was promised; who shut the mouths of lions, 34quenched the fury of the flames, and escaped the edge of the sword; whose weakness was turned to strength; and who became powerful in battle and routed foreign armies. 35Women received back their dead, raised to life again. Others were tortured and refused to be released, so that they might gain a better resurrection. 36Some faced jeers and flogging, while still others were chained and put in prison. 37They were stoned; they were sawed in two; they were put to death by the sword. They went about in sheepskins and goatskins, destitute, persecuted and mistreated— 38the world was not worthy of them. They wandered in deserts and mountains, and in caves and holes in the ground.

39These were all commended for their faith, yet none of them received what had been promised. 40God had planned something better for us so that only together with us would they be made perfect.

INSIGHTS ON HEALING

1. Reflect on this chapter and write down some of the kinds of obstacles that were overcome by faith in God.

2. Think for a moment about a circumstance in your life that seems impossible. What encouragement in these verses speaks to your situation?

3. Verse 39 tells us these heroes didn't receive all what had been promised because they died before Christ came. Living on this side of the Cross is a blessing we often forget. Pick one of the heroes mentioned and do a deeper study on their life. What acts of faith did they have to exercise? What were the outcomes of their obedience to believe in God to provide what they needed?

HEALING ENCOUNTER

I have a friend, Chauncy Crandall, who is a gifted heart specialist. Well, he has witnessed God raising two people from the dead through praying for the sick. I love him because he is so simple and matter-of-fact about his faith.

He told me he spoke to a group of doctors in Rome, 250 physicians, about heart conditions. Later in his presentation he asked them, "Now, would you like to hear how the name of Jesus heals?" He went on to challenge them with this question: "How many of you would like to be healed?" A group of doctors stood up, then *clunk*. A man in the front row began to fall. Then another in the back.

Chauncy said to me, "Marilyn, it was crazy. Doctors were falling all over the place by the power of the Spirit." Then one of the leading men who organized the conference came to talk to him; he was from Argentina.

"I'm having a medical conference in my country. Would you come and speak, Doctor?"

It's amazing how God is using Chauncy and his simple faith and simple prayers. He is amazed to see the dead rise because Jesus is answering prayers! We really have a big God and I'm praying that this study will make God bigger in your mind and heart, to ask of Him things you wouldn't ask.

"Father, I thank you for boldness to pray in the name of Jesus.
Thank you for the healing you provided for us at the Cross. Give us the courage to ask you to heal our friends, our family, and all those
you place in our paths. In Jesus' Name, Amen."

HEALING ACTION POINT/SECTION REVIEW

I trust this study is impacting your prayer life and that you feel more qualified to pray for the sick than you maybe thought was possible. Prayerfully walk through this Section Review Exercise before moving on to Section 2 of the syllabus.

1. Summarize in a few sentences what you've learned about God the Healer.

___

2. What key points do you want to remember about receiving your healing that have been discussed?

___

3. Write out Marilyn's simple definition of faith here.

4. Share with your group one praise from your prayer journal. If you are studying independently, write it out here and take a moment to give thanks.

section 2

KEEP YOUR HEALING

CHAPTER SIX

DON'T LET GO

"What do you conspire against the LORD? He will make an utter end of it. Affliction will not rise up a second time" (Nahum 1:9, NKJV).

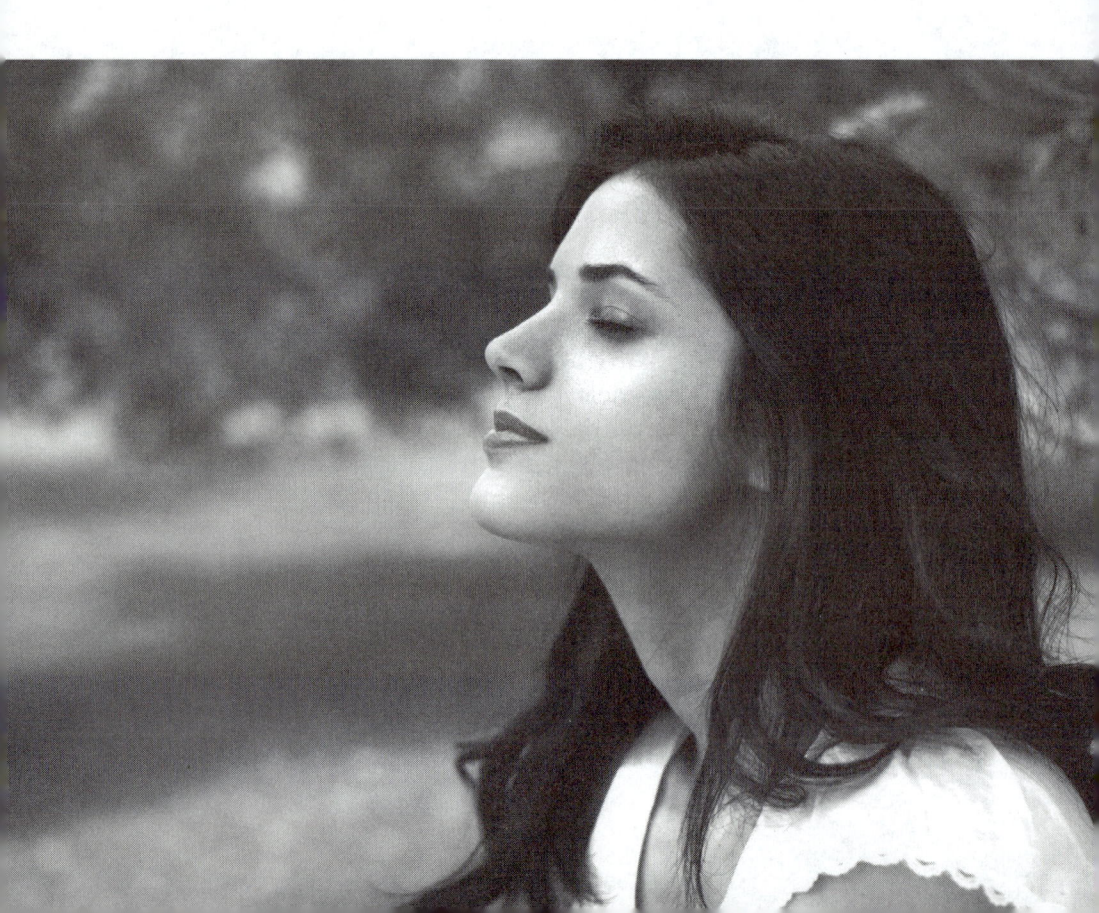

I've mentioned that healing can be a process and often is what we experience to be true. When a friend or family member hears a fatal diagnosis, sometimes it is hard to move out of that shock toward God. And that is an important step, to move toward God, not away.

I want to reference a powerful story of perseverance. Some dear friends, Kim and Bob Hritz, faced a battle with bone marrow cancer. You can imagine the devastation they felt. Before the test results came back from a normal check up, Bob was living life normally, feeling fine, and loving God and his family. His first thoughts, "God can't let this happen to us." Kim worked as an oncology nurse and God used all that knowledge she had in this serious battle they faced together. Yet in the end it wasn't just the medical knowledge or the procedures themselves that healed Bob. Their faith in God took them beyond the diagnosis toward the healing power of Jesus. There were rebounds, bad days, and discouraging reports they had to live through, but ultimately God gave them strength to fight and in the midst of the fight, they praised Him, and God did a miracle on Bob's behalf. In their book, The Good Fight: Our Battle with Cancer, the Hritz family shares the process and the determination God gave them to not let go of life.

Perhaps you are someone who has experienced God's healing touch, to find a symptom or the actual illness has come back. It's important we do not let the enemy steal what God has meant for you to have.

WORDS OF HEALING
TEXT: John 5:1-15 (NIV)

The Healing Pool

1Some time later, Jesus went up to Jerusalem for a feast of the Jews. 2Now there is in Jerusalem near the Sheep Gate a pool, which in Aramaic is called Bethesda and which is surrounded by five covered colonnades. 3-4Here a great number of disabled people used to lie—the blind, the lame, the paralyzed 5One who was there had been an invalid for thirty-eight years. 6When Jesus saw him lying there and learned that he had been in this condition for a long time, he asked him, "Do you want to get well?"
7"Sir," the invalid replied, "I have no one to help me into the pool when the water is stirred. While I am trying to get in, someone else goes down ahead of me."
8Then Jesus said to him, "Get up! Pick up your mat and walk." 9At once the man was cured; he picked up his mat and walked. The day on which this took place was a Sabbath, 10and so the Jews said to the man who had been healed, "It is the Sabbath; the law forbids you to carry your mat."
11But he replied, "The man who made me well said to me, 'Pick up your mat and walk.'"
12So they asked him, "Who is this fellow who told you to pick it up and walk?"
13The man who was healed had no idea who it was, for Jesus had slipped away into the crowd that was there.
14Later Jesus found him at the temple and said to him, "See, you are well again. Stop sinning or something worse may happen to you." 15The man went away and told the Jews that it was Jesus who had made him well.

INSIGHTS ON HEALING

1. Note how many years the man had been lame. What attitudes do you think the lame man might have struggled with for so many years? How do you feel trapped?

2. Describe a hardship that has caused you to lose hope in a certain area of your life.

3. In verse 14, what are Jesus' instructions to the man? Jesus does not hold that disease and sickness are always a result of personal sin. However there are times when we do have a role in our sickness. What are some sinful attitudes that you personally struggle with?

Sometimes we hear people say, "The devil made me do it." Well, the devil very well might have dropped wrong attitudes in your mind, but you have a choice in how you respond. I want to discuss some of the ways we can lose our healing from God. Sometimes the devil is scheming to steal it away and unfortunately there are ways we give him an advantage, a foothold, and much has to do with our attitudes!

"... and do not give the devil a foothold" (Ephesians 4:27, NIV).

Ephesians 4 lists some ways that we are not to live. Paul tells us to not let unwholesome talk come out of our mouths, to not be bitter, to refrain from slander and malice. The way we live our lives can actually make the Holy Spirit sad and the enemy has studied human nature long enough to know how to make our attitudes a place of weakness in our lives. The enemy wants us to stumble in two ways: One, through ungodly acts, and two, through ungodly attitudes.

Ungodly living takes its toll on our body, spirit, and mind. Now with this, we know God can heal anyone He chooses to heal—it can be the worst of sinners. Sometimes healing comes though someone is living completely at odds with God. However, Scripture tells us as believers, we are a new creation. The old has passed, the new has come. With that, we know that our lives should be committed to godly living. We need to protect our mind, our heart, and our bodies so that we are in a position to keep our healing—not be vulnerable to the enemy's schemes against us.

What about our attitudes? For some of us, our attitudes might be harder to control than succumbing to other temptations. It's easy to speak wrong words and sometimes we don't realize how they are affecting our lives. Words really do have power for life or death according to King Solomon, the wisest man in the Bible: "A fool finds no pleasure in understanding but delights in airing his own opinions" (Proverbs 18:2, NKJV). I believe our words do matter to God. What do our words say about what is in our hearts? Proverbs also tells us that out of our mouth, the heart speaks. The things we say can expose our attitudes and perspectives that are not healthy.

I want to share something that is almost too hard for our minds to grasp, but let me tell you of my own personal experience. I have more energy and more strength in my 70s-early 80s than I had in my twenties. When I was in my twenties, I was always whining and complaining about being tired.

My husband would come home and ask, "How are you?" My stock answer was, "I'm so tired!" Because Wally got so tired of hearing those words, he said my theme song was, "I'm Tired." He would really irritate me by singing to me an old song title "Tired, I'm So Tired." I wanted to slap him.

To be sure, teaching school and being a homemaker kept me busy. But that schedule didn't begin to compare with my schedule today, and now I'm full of energy!

What is the difference? In those days I was living life under the sun. I did not know how to live life under the Son; I didn't even know that kind of life was available. When I heard about the quality of life I could have in Christ, I began to appropriate that life. You know, Christians shouldn't just be looking for healing; we should be expecting divine health.

HEALING ENCOUNTER

He [God] said, *"If you listen carefully to the voice of the LORD your God and do what is right in his eyes, if you pay attention to his commands and keep all his decrees, I will not bring on you any of the diseases I brought on the Egyptians, for I am the LORD, who heals you"* (Exodus 15:26, NIV).

I want to point this verse out to you because it is the first time God refers to Himself as Healer. And because He is the God who heals, He wants to keep us healthy. Moses was the first one to reveal God as Healer. That is quite a revelation to share. And how hard it must have been for Moses to get the Israelites to grab onto that truth. The grumbling Israelites had examples to pull from to show Moses, "Well then why did this happen and why ...." Sometimes, you may find yourself alone in your conviction, but God asks you to look beyond the circumstances.

I share openly that I love and appreciate doctors—we need them and I don't tell people at all to stop going to them. Some Christians have been made to feel guilty for going to a doctor and taught it is a lack of faith. This is not my sentiment at all. However, I want to share a story about a family who grew up with no access to doctors. The mother, though, believed in praying for the health and wellness of her family. There were six children and the father was a Pentecostal pastor. They were radicals and, you know, probably worshiped in loud ways and perhaps some would think of them as naïve. Well they moved every year, from city to city—that is just what Church of God of Prophecy pastors had to do without questioning the overseers of the church. They simply did it.

This family was very poor and the children never went to a doctor until they were in their twenties. But they had a wonderful resource—their mother strongly believed in God's healing power. If something went wrong with their teeth, they got a cold, they had a fever, they just prayed. Today all six children and all the grandchildren are serving God. They aren't bitter they grew up poor and deprived, rather they are grateful for God somehow meeting their needs and protecting their health.

HEALING ACTION POINT

Write down all your questions about praying for healing. See if you can find the answers to your questions in God's Word. Use this as a group exercise and see of your group can discuss and answer together.

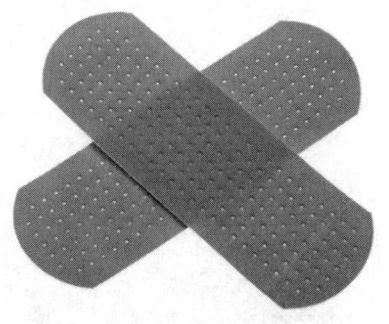

Notes:

CHAPTER SEVEN

HOW CAN I KEEP SOMETHING I HAVEN'T RECEIVED?

When Jesus saw their faith, he said, "Friend, your sins are forgiven" (Luke 5:20, NIV).

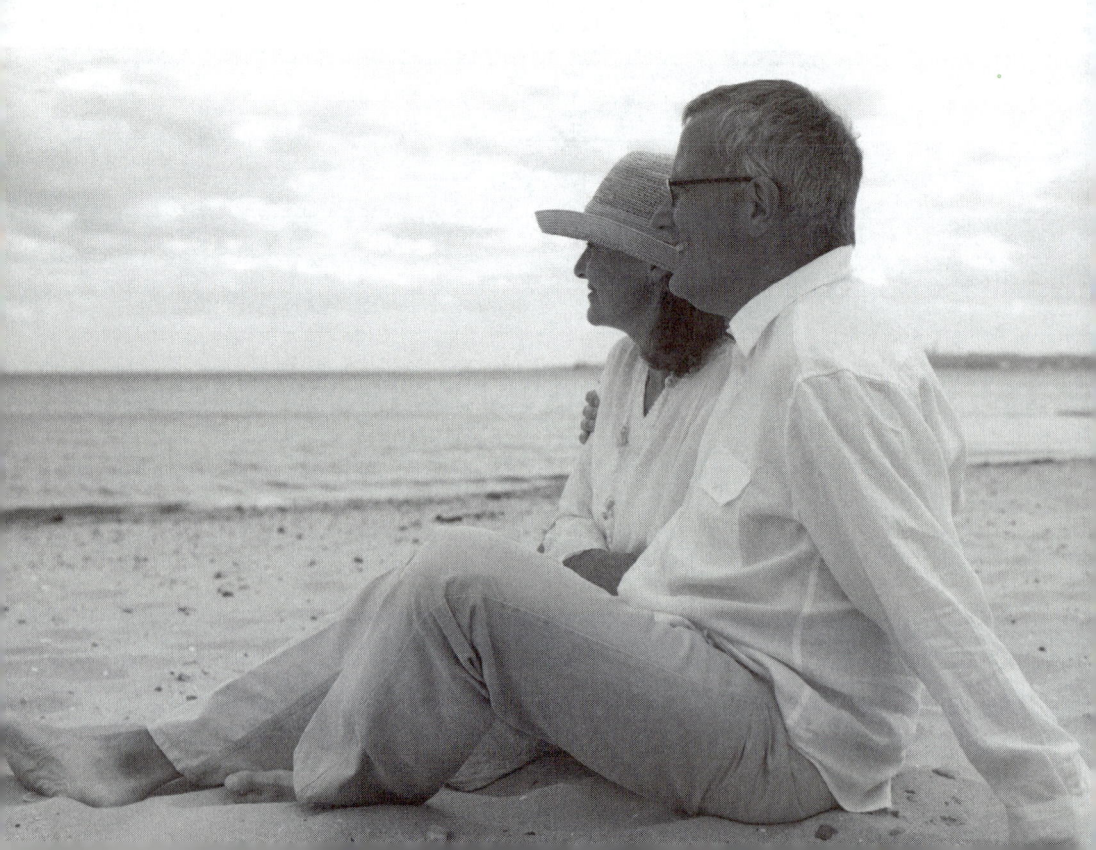

As we go through our study together, I want to be clear on something: I do not have all the answers as to why some are healed so quickly, yet others are not made well this side of heaven, no matter how much faith was present. You know, I've felt burdens to pray for people and gone to the hospital, only to get a hard phone call that they didn't pull through. We do have to sometimes appeal to mystery and to God's sovereignty. He knows all things and circumstances.

So meanwhile, we have to fight the good fight together and lean on one another when we've lost sight of what God can do. There are times in life when the faith of another is God's grace in our lives. We see this demonstrated in a story of healing found in Luke 5.

WORDS OF HEALING
Text: Luke 5:17-26 (NIV)

Healing of the Paralytic Man

17 One day as he was teaching, Pharisees and teachers of the law, who had come from every village of Galilee and from Judea and Jerusalem, were sitting there. And the power of the LORD was present for him to heal the sick. 18 Some men came carrying a paralytic on a mat and tried to take him into the house to lay him before Jesus. 19 When they could not find a way to do this because of the crowd, they went up on the roof and lowered him on his mat through the tiles into the middle of the crowd, right in front of Jesus.
20 When Jesus saw their faith, he said, "Friend, your sins are forgiven."
21 The Pharisees and the teachers of the law began thinking to themselves, "Who is this fellow who speaks blasphemy? Who can forgive sins but God alone?"
22 Jesus knew what they were thinking and asked, "Why are you thinking these things in your hearts? 23 Which is easier: to say, 'Your sins are forgiven,' or to say, 'Get up and walk'? 24 But that you may know that the Son of Man has authority on earth to forgive sins...." He said to the paralyzed man, "I tell you, get up, take your mat and go home." 25 Immediately he stood up in front of them, took what he had been lying on and went home praising God. 26 Everyone was amazed and gave praise to God. They were filled with awe and said, "We have seen remarkable things today."

In this story we see the love of faithful friends and how sometimes we rely on others to come to our side and walk with us when perhaps we cannot even walk ourselves. We all need the faith of others around us and the Body of Christ can be a place of healing for us. Maybe you are struggling with waiting for God to heal you and so you are afraid to keep praying and believing, thinking maybe you should give up. Lean on the faith of your friends!

INSIGHTS ON HEALING

1. Think of a time when you couldn't pray for yourself or your own faith was weak. How did God provide for you during that difficult time?

2. In many accounts of Jesus' healing ministry, we see the resistance from religious leaders. Can you speculate why the church seems afraid or resistant to talk about God as Healer during our corporate worship?

3. The friends in this passage were true friends. They believed that Jesus could heal their friend and they weren't going to let anything prevent them from getting to Jesus. Sometimes we don't help someone else because it means some kind of sacrifice for us. After reading this passage, pray and reflect if you feel like you are to allow someone else to borrow your faith, even it if requires extra effort from your end.

HEALING ACTION POINT

If you are going through this study as a small group or at church, schedule a time to take communion together. Be reminded that we are family and we share one another's burdens. There is a special Grace present when we remember together His sacrifice. And healing happens during communion, I believe, in special ways (see Appendix C for an outline of Scripture and service details).

After the communion service, record any miracles or insights you want to note in your prayer journal.

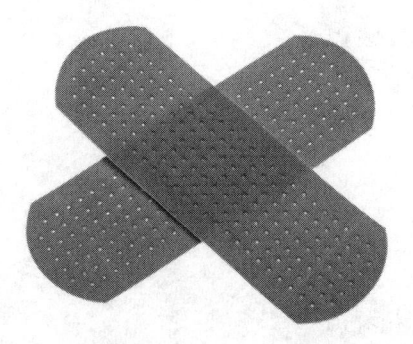

CHAPTER EIGHT

THE THREAT OF A STORM

"Others went out on the sea in ships; they were merchants on the mighty waters. They saw the works of the LORD, his wonderful deeds in the deep. For he spoke and stirred up a tempest that lifted high the waves. They mounted up to the heavens and went down to the depths; in their peril their courage melted away. They reeled and staggered like drunken men; they were at their wits' end. Then they cried out to the LORD in their trouble, and he brought them out of their distress" (Psalm 107:23-28, NIV).

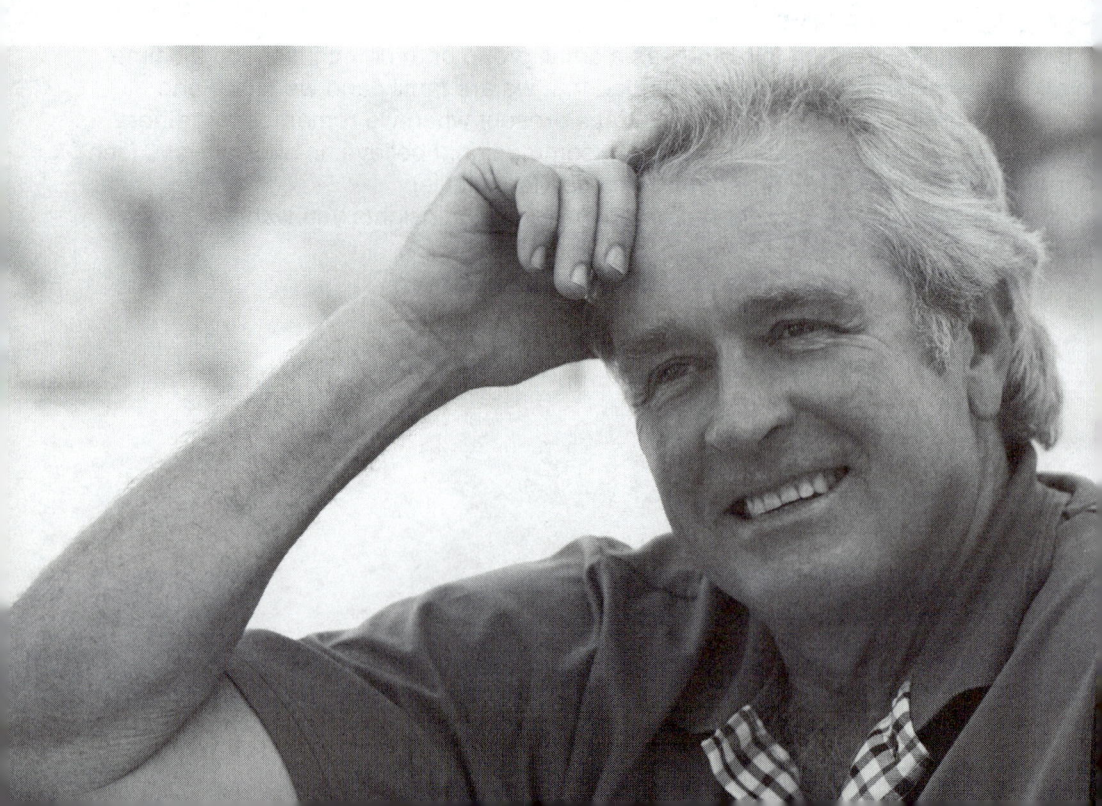

Storms hit our lives in all sorts of ways and it isn't always easy at first to discern the cause. However, I want to make this important point: Because you are in a storm right now does not mean it is because you are out of the will of God. Looking at the life of the Apostle Paul, we know he was faithful to follow God's lead. Yet often when he followed the Spirit, he was faced with real, honest hardships. And, literally, storms that left him shipwrecked. When Paul tells us about his floggings, starvation, sickness, dangers, and the enemies who came against him, it is clearly miraculous he survived.

Storms can prove to be a catalyst toward the ultimate will of God, but sometimes we become so focused on ourselves that we forget to see God is with us in the storm. In light of our discussion on healing, the enemy wants to keep you defeated, so he wants you to believe the storm is more powerful than God. And sometimes we succumb to unbelief. The most damaging thing that a storm can do is rob you of your faith in God. We often look for God once the storm is over but He asks us to keep our eyes on Him when things are at their worst.

Sometimes Paul was in a storm because he was right in the center of God's will. The Holy Spirit had directed Him to go to Rome (Acts 19:21). But he faced oppositions of every kind because he submitted his life to God. In Acts 27, we learn Paul experienced some hardships because others did not heed the guidance of God. But clearly, despite the disobedience of others, God protected them. He never abandons us in a storm. Taking care of us in a storm is God's specialty. He is our anchor when it feels like we can't even see where to turn. As you pray for healing for yourself and for others, it doesn't matter if you are in a storm or not. We have to keep our faith intact, so here are some reminders.

WHAT TO DO IN A STORM

1. Pray and Fast
2. Listen to God
3. Be Certain You Are With Faithful People
4. Encourage Yourself

WORDS OF HEALING
TEXT: Acts 27:1-44 (NIV)

Paul Sails for Rome
1When it was decided that we would sail for Italy, Paul and some other prisoners were handed over to a centurion named Julius, who belonged to the Imperial Regiment. 2We boarded a ship from Adramyttium about to sail for ports along the coast of the province of Asia, and we put out to sea. Aristarchus, a Macedonian from Thessalonica, was with us.
3The next day we landed at Sidon; and Julius, in kindness to Paul, allowed him to go to his friends so they might provide for his needs. 4From there we put out to sea again and passed to the lee of Cyprus because the winds were against us. 5When we had sailed across the open sea off the coast of Cilicia and Pamphylia, we landed at Myra in Lycia. 6There the centurion found an Alexandrian ship sailing for Italy and put us on board. 7We made slow headway for many days and had difficulty arriving off Cnidus. When the wind did not allow us to hold our course, we sailed to the lee of Crete, opposite Salmone. 8We moved along the coast with difficulty and came to a place called Fair Havens, near the town of Lasea.
9Much time had been lost, and sailing had already become dangerous because by now it was after the Fast.[a] So Paul warned them, 10"Men, I can see that our voyage is going to be disastrous and bring great loss to ship and cargo, and to our own lives also." 11But the centurion, instead of listening to what Paul said, followed the advice of the pilot and of the owner of the ship. 12Since the harbor was unsuitable to winter in, the majority decided that we should sail on, hoping to reach Phoenix and winter there. This was a harbor in Crete, facing both southwest and northwest.

The Storm
13When a gentle south wind began to blow, they thought they had obtained what they wanted; so they weighed anchor and sailed along the shore of Crete. 14Before very long, a wind of hurricane force, called the "northeaster," swept down from the island. 15The ship was caught by the storm and could not head into the wind; so we gave way to it and were driven along. 16As we passed to the lee of a small island called Cauda, we were hardly able to make the lifeboat secure. 17When the men had hoisted it aboard, they passed ropes under the ship itself to hold it together. Fearing that they would run aground on the sandbars of Syrtis, they lowered the sea anchor and let the ship be driven along. 18We took such a violent battering from the storm that the next day they began to throw the cargo overboard. 19On the third day, they threw the ship's tackle overboard with their own hands. 20When neither sun nor stars appeared for many days and the storm continued raging, we finally gave up all hope of being saved.
21After the men had gone a long time without food, Paul stood up before them and said: "Men, you should have taken my advice not to sail from Crete; then you would have spared yourselves this damage and loss. 22But now I urge you to keep up your courage, because not one of you will be lost; only the ship will be destroyed. 23Last night an angel of the God whose I am and whom I serve stood beside me 24and said, 'Do not be afraid, Paul. You must stand trial before Caesar; and God has graciously

given you the lives of all who sail with you.' ₂₅So keep up your courage, men, for I have faith in God that it will happen just as he told me. ₂₆Nevertheless, we must run aground on some island."

The Shipwreck

₂₇On the fourteenth night we were still being driven across the Adriatic Sea, when about midnight the sailors sensed they were approaching land. ₂₈They took soundings and found that the water was a hundred and twenty feet deep. A short time later they took soundings again and found it was ninety feet deep. ₂₉Fearing that we would be dashed against the rocks, they dropped four anchors from the stern and prayed for daylight. ₃₀In an attempt to escape from the ship, the sailors let the lifeboat down into the sea, pretending they were going to lower some anchors from the bow. ₃₁Then Paul said to the centurion and the soldiers, "Unless these men stay with the ship, you cannot be saved." ₃₂So the soldiers cut the ropes that held the lifeboat and let it fall away.

₃₃Just before dawn Paul urged them all to eat. "For the last fourteen days," he said, "you have been in constant suspense and have gone without food—you haven't eaten anything. ₃₄Now I urge you to take some food. You need it to survive. Not one of you will lose a single hair from his head." ₃₅After he said this, he took some bread and gave thanks to God in front of them all. Then he broke it and began to eat. ₃₆They were all encouraged and ate some food themselves. ₃₇Altogether there were 276 of us on board. ₃₈When they had eaten as much as they wanted, they lightened the ship by throwing the grain into the sea.

₃₉When daylight came, they did not recognize the land, but they saw a bay with a sandy beach, where they decided to run the ship aground if they could. ₄₀Cutting loose the anchors, they left them in the sea and at the same time untied the ropes that held the rudders. Then they hoisted the foresail to the wind and made for the beach. ₄₁But the ship struck a sandbar and ran aground. The bow stuck fast and would not move, and the stern was broken to pieces by the pounding of the surf.

₄₂The soldiers planned to kill the prisoners to prevent any of them from swimming away and escaping. ₄₃But the centurion wanted to spare Paul's life and kept them from carrying out their plan. He ordered those who could swim to jump overboard first and get to land. ₄₄The rest were to get there on planks or on pieces of the ship. In this way everyone reached land in safety.

INSIGHTS ON HEALING

1. Storms can overtake our lives, so much so, we just ride the waves as Paul did—until the sun comes out. What were some of Paul's reactions to this particular storm?

2. Sometimes when we are in a storm God still calls us to encourage others. Paul was doing just that as well, sharing his faith with others when those aboard the ship were afraid. He was even comforting those who did not follow his advice. Think about someone God may be asking you to encourage through reaching out to them or praying for their healing and comfort, even though you may not agree on everything, or you yourself may be hurting.

"For I will restore health to you and heal you of your wounds" (Jeremiah 30:17, NKJV).

3. The last verse in the chapter says, "everyone reached land in safety." Take a moment and reflect on a storm you have been through in the past and how God proved faithful. What did you learn about God in the midst of the storm? What things did you conclude once you had been through it?

_____
_____
_____
_____
_____
_____
_____
_____
_____
_____
_____
_____
_____

HEALING ENCOUNTER

We often have to be willing to fight a battle to get and keep our healing. I heard of a faithful pastor who was in the middle of purchasing a building for his house of worship. The building was in foreclosure and he knew it was being occupied by a drug ring. Well, one night some thugs came to his door a week before Christmas. The voice outside stated they were UPS, so he didn't think that was unusual, though it was around 11:30 pm.

When the pastor opened the door, two men beat him to the ground with a lead pipe, threatening him, "Give up the building." The pastor became unconscious and later found himself in a hospital bed with 40 stitches. God had spoken to him earlier that the building would be for his church and so he knew there was no way he could let go of that word from God.

The doctors told him it was a miracle he didn't suffer brain damage but to expect severe headaches and seizures. Well, his faithful mother was a woman of prayer and she asked for his healing, believing the blood of Jesus could heal him completely. The pastor didn't even have one headache and went on to occupy that building.

It's true sometimes storms come because we are holding on to what God spoke to us to do. Yet He is faithful to carry out His plan in the midst of the storm.

HEALING ACTION POINT

1. Identify two crises in your life right now. If you do not have one, think of someone close to you in the midst of a real storm.

2. Define two miracles needed for each crisis.

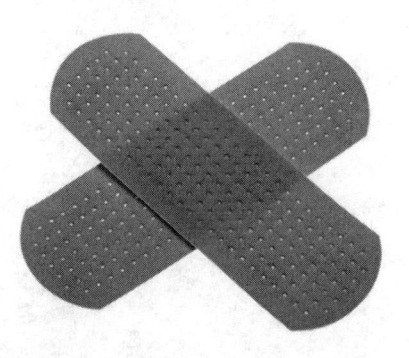

Notes:

CHAPTER NINE

FIGHT THE GOOD FIGHT

"Fight the good fight of the faith. Take hold of the eternal life to which you were called when you made your good confession in the presence of many witnesses" (1 Timothy 6:12, NIV).

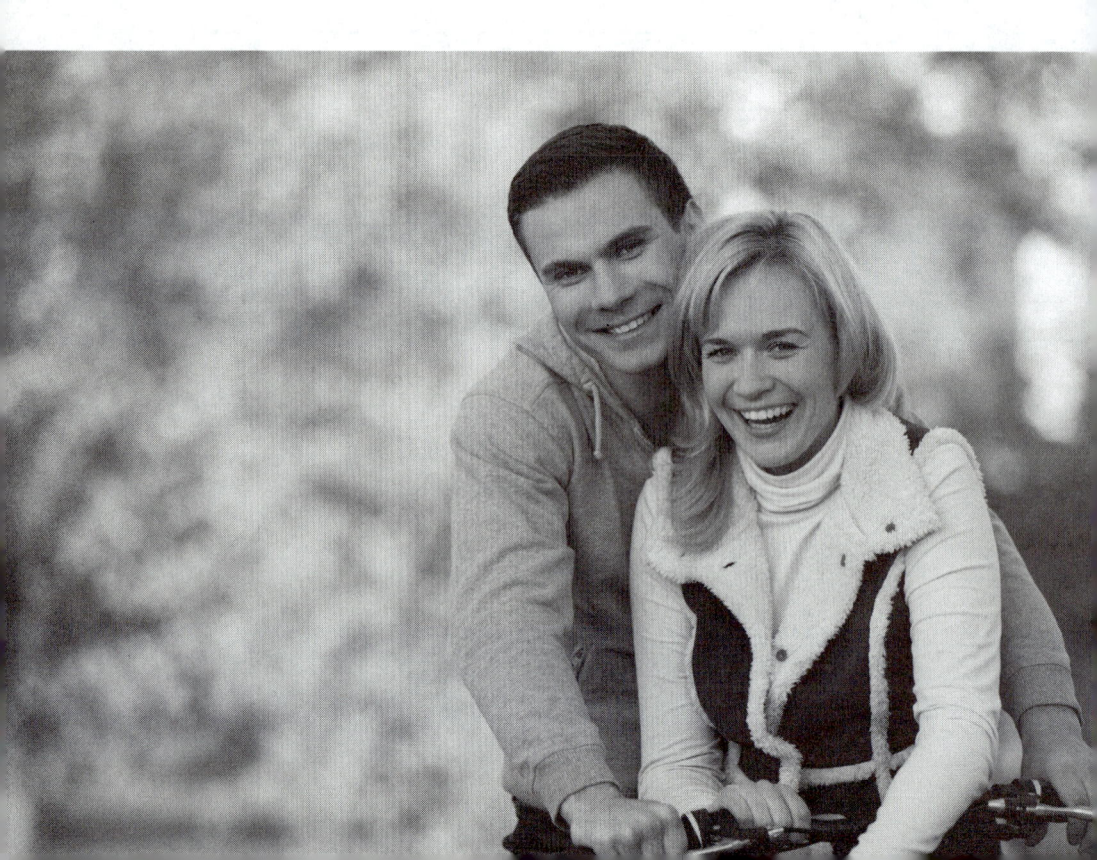

I will say it again here—you have to fight for your health. We are in a battle to receive and to keep our healing in this life. We know the enemy wants to destroy our families, our homes, and our churches. He does not want us to experience the blessings of God. He does not want us to acknowledge that God is a good, loving LORD.

The enemy wants us to just give up and not fight the good fight. We know we aren't alone in the fight, that God is present with us in all situations, but that doesn't mean fighting isn't hard. Years ago a well-known pastor lost a battle with cancer, but a personal friend of his told me that this pastor wanted to go home to be with his God. So in a sense, you could say he was not in the mindset to fight and he was ready to move on from this life. So we do have a level of input, so it seems. You've heard of those who have decided to hang on until a loved one arrives so they can say goodbye. Once that person comes, they have a peace to let go and give up their spirit.

It isn't always easy to discern why some die and some recover. Some die because they are in the realm of fear and doubt, and some die because they are not protecting their soul and live in harm's way. Still others die, and none of us this side of eternity will ever know why; but we don't quit trusting God. Job had no idea that it was Satan who brought all his trouble, but he could still say of God, "Though He slay me, yet I will trust him..." (Job 13:15).

We can't deny that people who receive prayer for healing are not always healed; they may even die. I don't have all the answers and neither does any other person, but I'm not going to stop praying and believing the LORD will touch people with His healing power. If I am praying for someone at a church service and just a few are healed, I'll still keep praying for the sick. It is a biblical thing to do. Don't ever allow what looks like defeat dampen your zeal to pray a healing prayer for yourself and others. James 5:15 says the prayer of faith will save the sick and the LORD will raise them up.

KEEP RIGHT RELATIONSHIPS

The most important aspect of life is relationships because of the eternal value. It is hard to see the breakdown of the family continue to be the norm as we see so many marriages ending in divorce. I've heard many confess, I gave up on the fight too soon. We want to say so often, "It just isn't worth it." But, your family is always worth it! You may be convinced there is no way God could ever heal your marriage or your family. That is something that is contrary to what Scripture teaches us. God knows all the pain, misunderstandings, or generational curses that are involved. But He can heal any rift in a relationship if we fight for what God wants us to have, and most of the time a process is involved.

My mother was an Irish-French woman who was born and bred in Texoma—and had a faith as big as Texas. I grew up with Methodist roots, but more on the liberal side of the denomination. I don't remember hearing much about the Bible in our church growing up. Yet, God had a firm hand on my family.

While my father provided for us, and we always had food and shelter, he struggled with a mental illness and was quite abusive to my mother. Mother was the parent who kept us all going, who encouraged us, and who provided the stability my brother

David and I needed.

The LORD became more real to me when I witnessed His power right in my home. When I was about 19, my Mom started going to a charismatic church—very different from our Methodist upbringing. I didn't care for it much, but I didn't complain about it. My mom would ask me to come with her on Sundays, and I thought they were way too emotional, too loud. I didn't like hearing people speak in tongues and was skeptical about all of their noisy worship. But during this time, I noticed Mother had a new confidence about her faith, which my father also noticed. He hated her new church and became more verbally abusive the more involved she became.

"Mary, if you go to that church one more time, I'll kill you!" he hissed. But Mother continued to go faithfully, despite his disapproval. Then the day came that I feared most.

"Marilyn, where is your mother?"

I knew she was at church, but I replied back to my father, "I don't know," trying to look as unruffled as possible. A couple of hours later, Mom came home and he grabbed a knife as he heard her come in the back door.

"Have you been at church?" he intoned with the knife poised.

"In the name of Jesus, you drop that knife!"

I saw my father shrink to the floor, completely overpowered by the Spirit. I witnessed the power of God protect my Mom with my own eyes. Peace flooded the room. I knew my father couldn't harm her, and my fear ceased.

"John, I will continue to be a good wife, cook, clean, and do your laundry. But I will also continue to go to church three times a week."

He was unable to move for quite a while, though I'm not sure how long it was. I had never witnessed anything like that before, but I knew God was at work. He became more relevant to me, more traceable even in the small things, after that encounter. And you know what? My dad was healed later from his mental illness because he had family who were praying and who were fighting for healthy relationships!

STAY IN CHURCH

Being a pastor's wife, I've been so blessed to have strong families of faith surround my own. I also have seen people come and go and give up on their church, ending up alone, unprotected spiritually.

We live in such an age of individuality. And it is easy to justify why we stopped going to this church or that church. But there is a reason Scripture says: "Let us hold fast the confession of our hope without wavering, for He who promised is faithful. And let us consider one another in order to stir up love and good works, not forsaking the assembling of ourselves together, as is the manner of some, but exhorting one another, and so much the more as you see the Day approaching" (Hebrews 10:23-25, NKJV).

There is no perfect church because we are all imperfect. There have been grave abuses done in the name of the church, but Jesus loved the church so much He died for her. Our mandate is to love the body of Christ as He did. The enemy knows that the worst witness of the church is our dividedness. That's why I feel so blessed to have Catholic friends, Methodist friends, Baptist friends—we all need each other. You were never meant to work your faith alone.

If you have not committed to one local church, I pray that during this study God would lead you to a sound, healthy church where you can grow and be supported. This will help you be able to continue to fight the good fight more effectively.

CRUCIFY THE FLESH

The Apostle Paul understood how hard it was to follow Jesus. When we are tired it is easy to make wrong choices, because we aren't willing to say no to our flesh. It is a battle that we must engage.

We have never been promised an easy road. Jesus said to be a disciple we had to deny self and pick up our cross in order to follow Him. In Romans 7, we hear about Paul's honest struggle to make the right choices. He didn't understand why he would end up doing exactly what he didn't want to do. When we allow our flesh to rule our decisions, we can become trapped and unable to do the will of God. Our flesh can keep us from fighting the battle, from staying committed to a church, or from mending broken relationships. Once we realize where we are vulnerable, it will be so much easier to believe God does want to heal us, that He is hearing our prayers.

WORDS OF HEALING
TEXT: Romans 7:14-25 (NIV)

Struggling

14 We know that the law is spiritual; but I am unspiritual, sold as a slave to sin. 15 I do not understand what I do. For what I want to do I do not do, but what I hate I do. 16 And if I do what I do not want to do, I agree that the law is good. 17 As it is, it is no longer I myself who do it, but it is sin living in me. 18 I know that nothing good lives in me, that is, in my sinful nature.[c] For I have the desire to do what is good, but I cannot carry it out. 19 For what I do is not the good I want to do; no, the evil I do not want to do—this I keep on doing. 20 Now if I do what I do not want to do, it is no longer I who do it, but it is sin living in me that does it.
21 So I find this law at work: When I want to do good, evil is right there with me. 22 For in my inner being I delight in God's law; 23 but I see another law at work in the members of my body, waging war against the law of my mind and making me a prisoner of the law of sin at work within my members. 24 What a wretched man I am! Who will rescue me from this body of death? 25 Thanks be to God—through Jesus Christ our Lord! So then, I myself in my mind am a slave to God's law, but in the sinful nature a slave to the law of sin.

INSIGHTS ON HEALING

1. Take a moment to identify a place in your life that may prevent you from fighting the good fight.

_____
_____
_____
_____
_____
_____
_____
_____
_____
_____

2. In Romans 7, Paul shows us the inner battle we face every day. Name some inner battles you are facing right now in your walk with God.

_____
_____
_____
_____
_____
_____
_____
_____
_____
_____
_____

3. You may know of someone who has a severe addiction and cannot let go. Take a moment to pray healing over them and for them to understand the power of God's grace. Pray a Scripture of healing over them (see Appendix B).

HEALING ENCOUNTER

I want to share with you the thrilling testimony of a woman who was healed of multiple sclerosis. She wrote, "I was finally able to let go of all the fears related to the MS which had kept me a prisoner for over 24 years. Thanks to God's love and the sacrifice of my precious Lord Jesus, I'm healed—I'm free!"

At the age of 16, this lady had been diagnosed with the disease that held her captive for over half her life. Then one day she told a friend she was sick and tired of being sick. Her friend began to open the healing Scriptures to her; and after some time, when the woman was convinced Jesus could heal her, the friend's sister prayed for the woman held so long in Satan's prison.

The letter said, "When my friend's sister laid hands on me and cast out the MS in the name of Jesus, I felt a warmth all through me. She touched various parts of my afflicted body, and I was a bit scared. Yet I felt a peace and calm when she finished.

The lady saw no immediate improvement, but she kept speaking the Word until she was able to accept her healing as done. From that moment the woman began to improve and today she is totally free from multiple sclerosis—glory to God! This lady wrote to me because during the time after she received prayer and the full manifestation of her healing, she received inspiration through some of my tapes.

Sometimes, we have to be patient and continue to believe God is at work.

HEALING ACTION POINT

Take a moment to write down a time when you felt like you had no strength to complete a difficult task, yet God gave you strength. It's important to remember such times so we are not tempted to miss opportunities to be used by God. You may want to pray this simple prayer as a way to make you more mindful of His plan for your day:

Lord, what is it that you want me to join you in doing today? Who can I touch and share my faith in you with as the Healer? Lead and guide my heart today and help me to be generous toward others. In Jesus' Name, Amen.

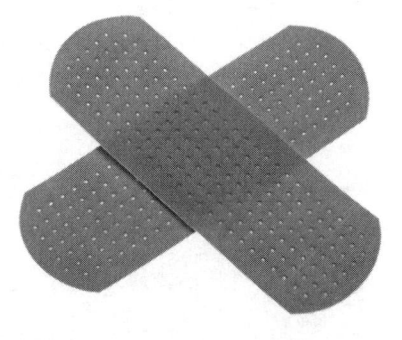

section 3

SICKNESS AND DEMONS

CHAPTER TEN

SICKNESS

"The thief cometh not, but for to steal, and to kill, and to destroy: I [Jesus] am come that that they might have life, and that they might have it more abundantly" (John 10:10, KJV).

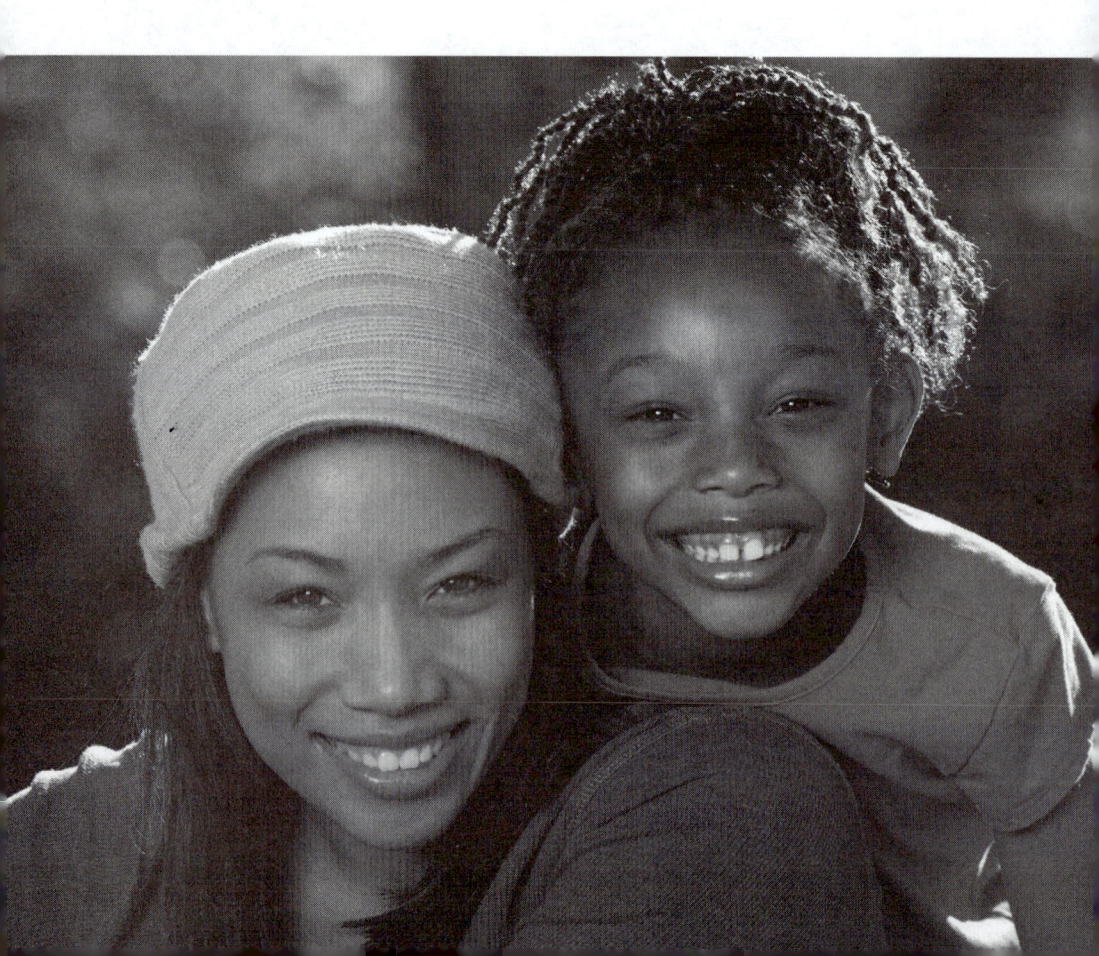

I get excited every time I see or hear a miracle of healing. You don't have to just read the Bible to experience encounters of healing. Whoever you are, wherever you are, you can experience His healing touch this very moment. You may be going through this teaching because you are asking for God to heal you. Or you may have a burden to pray for the healing of others. Even still, you may not be quite convinced that God is your healer. But I believe His Word can change our doubts that He does want us to ask and come to Him for our healing.

It's easy to become discouraged when a friend comes back from the doctor with news they have cancer. Perhaps you struggle with understanding why a child has to suffer with a terminal illness. I am someone who believes that the enemy wants us to be sick, to give up so we cannot share with others the power of Christ in our lives. In this whole discussion of healing, I think it is important to know when sickness began.

God made us in His image and His likeness. Since we know that God is good and everything He created is good, how did Satan and evil come into existence? Before creation, Lucifer decided he would lift his throne above God's throne and enlisted a third of the angels who rebelled with him. Of course, sin could not exist in the presence of God, so they were cast out of God's heaven (Isaiah 14:12-15; Ezekiel 28:12-19). When Lucifer should have been praising God, he made himself the center of pride and he fell.

But how did the devil set up shop on earth and become involved in sickness? How did he manage to make God's children sick in the first place? Well, the devil became the inflictor when humankind fell and sinned against God. Adam and Eve opened the door to sin, and sin opened the door to all of Satan's work. Before the Fall, there was no sickness or disease in the Garden of Eden. Adam and Eve were given eternal life. There was no death or dying before they sinned against God. Sickness is just an acceleration toward death.

I can honestly tell you I do feel even stronger in these years of life than I've felt at any other time. I do believe it is the covering of prayers of my community and also the Scriptures I speak out in the morning. So yes, I believe God can even take away sicknesses that are related to aging. It doesn't matter how old you are, healing is for all people. I believe sickness has a spiritual life. When Adam and Eve obeyed the devil, they disobeyed God and gave up their God-given authority over the earth. Their earthly blessings fell into the hands of the deceiver. And it's true with us, too:

"Don't you know that when you offer yourselves to someone to obey him as slaves, you are slaves to the one whom you obey—whether you are slaves to sin, which leads to death, or to obedience, which leads to righteousness?" (Romans 6:16, NIV)

The devil's plan was to make us a slave to sin and death, but then God sent Jesus to heal and redeem us. Every parent on earth, who knows the agony of seeing their children sick, has some idea of how God, our heavenly parent, must feel when we are diseased. Most parents would willingly take the illness of their children upon themselves rather than have their offspring ill. This is exactly what the Father did for us when Jesus went to the Cross and died for the sickness of sin. He redeemed us, and in that full redemption was the healing of your body.

"Because we have these promises, dear friends, let us cleanse ourselves from everything that can defile our body or spirit. And let us work toward complete holiness because we fear God" (2 Corinthians 7:1, NLT).

WORDS OF HEALING
TEXT: Isaiah 53; 1 Peter 2; Luke 13 (NIV)

Isaiah 53:4, 5
4 Surely he took up our infirmities
   and carried our sorrows,
   yet we considered him stricken by God,
   smitten by him, and afflicted.
5 But he was pierced for our transgressions,
   he was crushed for our iniquities;
   the punishment that brought us peace was upon him,
   and by his wounds we are healed.

1 Peter 2:24
He himself bore our sins in his body on the tree, so that we might die to sins and live for righteousness; by his wounds you have been healed.

Luke 13:10-17
10 On a Sabbath Jesus was teaching in one of the synagogues, 11 and a woman was there who had been crippled by a spirit for eighteen years. She was bent over and could not straighten up at all. 12 When Jesus saw her, he called her forward and said to her, "Woman, you are set free from your infirmity." 13 Then he put his hands on her, and immediately she straightened up and praised God.
14 Indignant because Jesus had healed on the Sabbath, the synagogue ruler said to the people, "There are six days for work. So come and be healed on those days, not on the Sabbath."
15 The LORD answered him, "You hypocrites! Doesn't each of you on the Sabbath untie his ox or donkey from the stall and lead it out to give it water? 16 Then should not this woman, a daughter of Abraham, whom Satan has kept bound for eighteen long years, be set free on the Sabbath day from what bound her?"
17 When he said this, all his opponents were humiliated, but the people were delighted with all the wonderful things he was doing.

INSIGHTS ON HEALING

1. There are those who believe God disciplines us with sickness, so we will go to Him. No doubt, God uses all things meant for evil for His good. That is the kind of God He is. In light of these Scriptures, what can we know about sickness, and what is Jesus' response to sickness?

2. What does Scripture say was the cause of the woman's illness in Luke 13? Read verses 11 and 16.

3. In the passage from Luke, Jesus rebukes the synagogue ruler for his indignant response to Him healing on the Sabbath. What religious rules have we imposed on Jesus today when it comes to our own healing?

HEALING ENCOUNTER

I go to a lot of churches that don't particularly emphasize healing and they really don't want me to pray for the sick. And course then, rebuking spirits, this makes people very nervous when you begin to deal with demons. When you are praying for healing, there will be times when God will have you rebuke the devil. But don't make a big deal out of it—the devil loves attention. Sometimes people will come up and give a big demonstration of a demon. But don't do that; don't let spirits take over. During a service, I've learned you don't need to give evil more attention than necessary. It doesn't need to take up a whole service. I don't let there be a display of a demonic fit—I just have the sick person leave the service. Demons don't have to be cast out in front of everybody. Jesus dealt with it always very quickly. He didn't belabor it and say, "What's your name. Where did you come from?"

The first time Wally and I dealt with demons, we did it all wrong. The lady was healed, not because of us, but because of the mercy of God. She picked our name out of the telephone book and we had just started our church. At the time, we had about sixty people and were eager to be available however God was leading.

"I'm having a nervous breakdown and I saw your name, your church ... would you come and pray for me?" she pleaded. I learned she was a 27-year-old mother with three little boys and had been in and out of a mental hospital.

We went to her and found her shaking. Wally spontaneously went over and knelt down and said, "In Jesus' name, I rebuke you Satan. The demon cried out of her and said, "I'm coming out of her into you."

At this time, I'm thinking, I'm leaving. It scared Wally too, but he said, "Well, what we do, Bonnie, is we are going to fast and pray for you. We're going to get some people in our church to intercede for ten days. Then we'll come back and pray with you." So we did.

We took her to a church to cast the demons out of her. We had a tape recorder. Now that is ridiculous—we even said we'd tape it so we could learn from what the demon said. Later, we realized, Well who learns from a demon? They are liars. Why would anyone listen to anything they had to say?

We were young in ministry so we didn't know better and asked, "What is your name? ... How many are in there? ... When did you come in?" We had at least four sessions, but she was still possessed and we were very frustrated.

There was a spirit-filled woman there who said, "Let me help you." Well she didn't play around at all. She didn't turn on the tape recorder. She just said, "Come out in Jesus' name." She took authority, but not by making a lot of noise or acting out in a lot of hype. And that was the end of that; Bonnie was delivered.

I learned, just don't mess around—cast them out and be done. Scripture shows that Jesus cast out spirits with the Word. Demons do move at the command of God's Word. Speak God's Word to them. That's what Jesus did.

HEALING ACTION POINT

Go to Appendix D and read over the Miracles of Jesus. Take time to read through them carefully and journal. Note how Jesus went about healing people. What were some of the things He asked people to do? Listen to the Spirit as your read over these and write out the things that stand out to you, though you may have read some of these miracles over and over before. Read with a fresh mind and heart.

Notes:

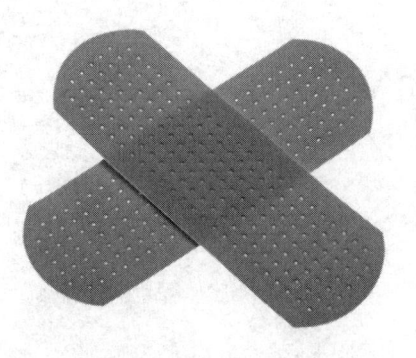

CHAPTER ELEVEN

DEMONS

I've been guilty of blaming the devil when I was really the one who needed to repent.
—Marilyn

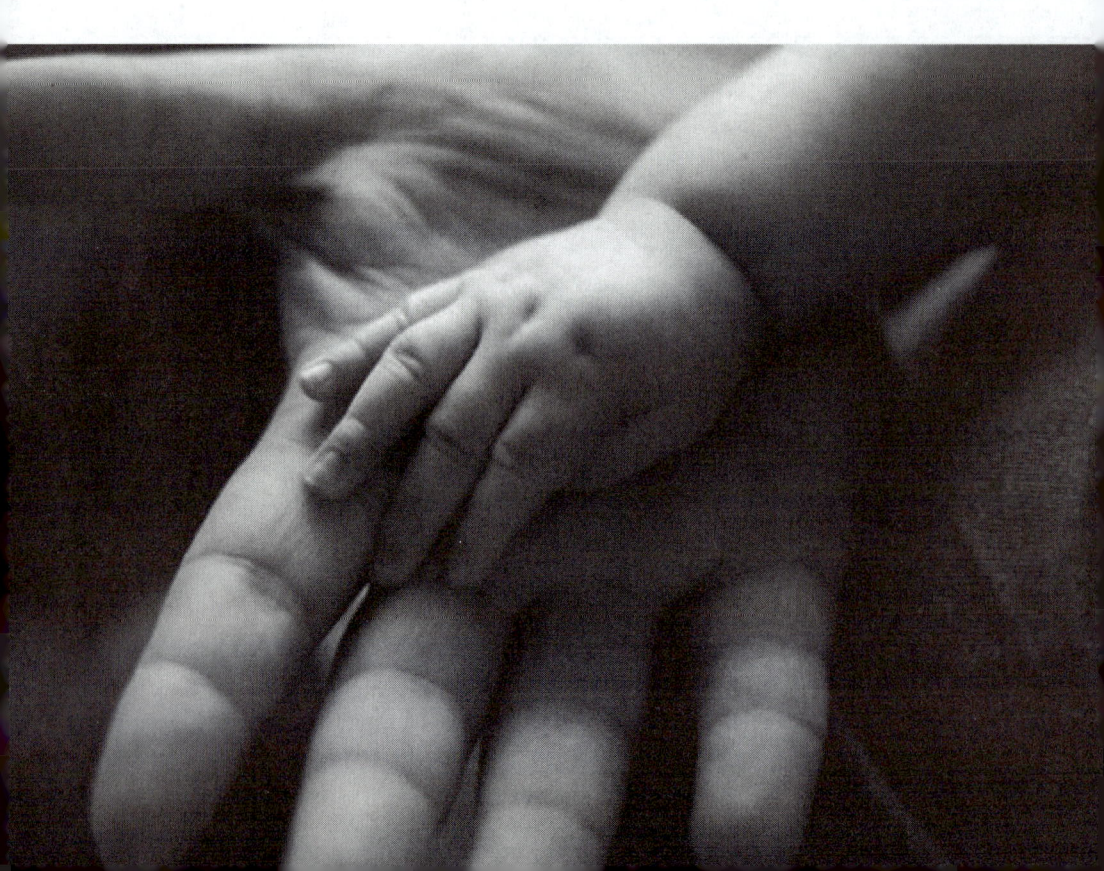

In chapter ten, I mentioned how important it is to not give too much attention to demons. This is a key point to grasp in this discussion. However, I do want to talk about them in regard to this whole topic of healing because they do cause sickness and disease, which all started with the curse of the Fall that Satan put on humanity. God explained what the curse would bring humans and that it came from Satan. So from there, the whole earth was out of kilter; it was under a curse. There is no doubt that sin brings sickness, disease, and everything that is unwhole (see 1 Thessalonians 5:23).

I am not saying that you have committed a sin every time you get sick. There are people who put a guilt trip on those who are ill by implying that their sickness is a result of some sin in their life. Remember, the Fall brought sickness and death and they are at work in our world. Babies are born with illnesses and these precious lives are not sick due to sin. Jesus Himself made it clear that it is not necessarily sin in an individual that causes their illness:

"And as Jesus passed by, he saw a man which was blind from his birth. And his disciples asked him, saying, Master, who did sin, this man, or his parents, that he was blind? Jesus answered, 'Neither has this man sinned, nor his parents ...'" (John 9:1-3).

Demons aren't always the cause either. I've been guilty of blaming the devil when I was really the one who needed to repent. I remember years ago I became angry over a situation. A certain person had pulled some bad business deals on people in our congregation. Although the matter had been handled, I began to meditate on it; and the more I meditated the angrier I became. Shortly after that I came down with severe flu symptoms: sore throat, temperature, chills. Of course I rebuked the devil—without results. Can you imagine how shocked I was when the LORD said, "The devil isn't the problem; you are." The LORD showed me how I had opened the door to sickness by allowing bitterness to lodge in my heart. What the person did was wrong but I needed to leave the matter with God. Needless to say, I repented of my sin and slammed the "door" on the sickness—and received my healing! Many times it is the devil and his demons who are the culprits, but sometimes it may even have to do with us.

Determining what to pray and how to pray for healing will be clear as you learn to listen to the Holy Spirit for guidance.

WORDS OF HEALING
TEXT: Luke 4:31-36 (NIV)

Jesus Drives Out an Evil Spirit

31 Then he went down to Capernaum, a town in Galilee, and on the Sabbath began to teach the people. 32 They were amazed at his teaching, because his message had authority.

33 In the synagogue there was a man possessed by a demon, an evil spirit. He cried out at the top of his voice, 34 "Ha! What do you want with us, Jesus of Nazareth? Have

you come to destroy us? I know who you are—the Holy One of God!"

35 "Be quiet!" Jesus said sternly. "Come out of him!" Then the demon threw the man down before them all and came out without injuring him.

36 All the people were amazed and said to each other, "What is this teaching? With authority and power he gives orders to evil spirits and they come out!"

TEXT: Matthew 8:14-17 (NIV)

Jesus Heals Many

14 When Jesus came into Peter's house, he saw Peter's mother-in-law lying in bed with a fever. 15 He touched her hand and the fever left her, and she got up and began to wait on him. 16 When evening came, many who were demon-possessed were brought to him, and he drove out the spirits with a word and healed all the sick. 17 This was to fulfill what was spoken through the prophet Isaiah: "He took up our infirmities and carried our diseases."

INSIGHTS ON HEALING

1. In Luke's account of healing, note how Jesus approached the healing of the demon-possessed man.

2. In Matthew, how did Jesus drive out the evil spirits?

3. Do you find it hard to believe that demons exist? How can we find the right balance in realizing they have influence, yet not give them too much attention?

HEALING ENCOUNTER

The first time I went to Kiev was right after the iron curtain fell down in Russia and the Ukraine. We wanted to see if we could come and have a healing meeting. I had a staff person with me to begin the planning process. When we got off of the plane a group of ORU students met us to drive us to the hotel where we were going to stay. The group approached me and said, "On your way to your hotel, would you mind casting a demon out of a girl we met?" Well, we had been on and off of planes for 24 hours, so I said, "Could it wait until tomorrow?"

One young man said to me, "No, no, we can't wait. We've been witnessing on the streets and we have got this girl to come and watch the Jesus film in Russian and she is there with her grandmother.

I asked him, "How do you know she is demon-possessed?" In my mind, I was thinking, how do these young students know what a demon is? A few of the students began to explain to me that she hears voices and cuts surfaces on her skin. They learned that she had been to a fortune teller and a curse was placed on her. They said she was bleeding but not from the demons cutting her. Well, from what they said, I knew they were right.

My flesh was wiped out. So, I said, "Lord, I'm tired. And He quickly said, "I'm not." I went into the room where Natasha was and saw her grandmother as well. She was about 16 years old and beautiful, yet pitiful. We gathered and it wasn't dramatic at all. We just prayed and took authority over the devil. When we did that, she fell to the floor, like she had fainted. But, when she got up, you could tell she was free. Her eyes and her whole face were different.

Well seven months later, I went back to have our meeting. When I got off the plane, there was Natasha. She had learned one sentence in English: "I love Jesus." And all her family became believers.

I was so glad I listened to God's strength, not my weakness.

"My flesh and my heart may fail, but God is the strength of my heart and my portion forever" (Psalm 73:26, NIV).

HEALING ACTION POINT

"They overcame him by the blood of the Lamb and by the word of their testimony; they did not love their lives so much as to shrink from death"
(Revelation 12:11, NIV).

There is something very powerful about the spoken word—and when we speak about what God has done for us, whether we are talking about a physical or a spiritual healing. Make it a point to share your testimony with someone in your study group or ask the LORD to show who to share your own testimony with.

section 4

HEALING THE SICK

CHAPTER TWELVE

THE POWER OF COMMUNITY

"But you have an anointing from the Holy One, and all of you know the truth..."
(1 John 2:20, NIV).

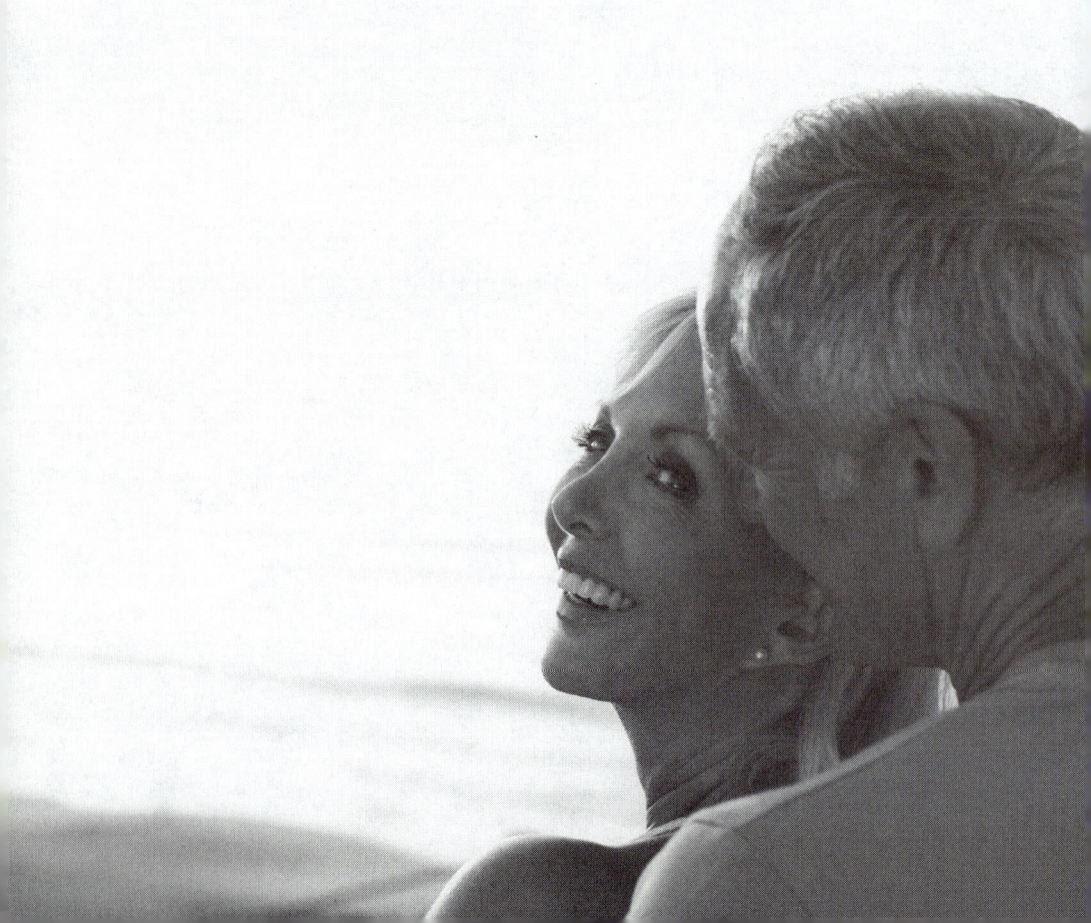

I love teaching on healing because I definitely believe we do not talk about it enough in corporate worship. Christianity is relational and when Jesus ascended after the resurrection, He gave us the gift of the Church and the gift of the Holy Spirit. We were meant to encourage one another, bear one another's burdens, and work out our faith together. It doesn't take long to figure out how the enemy hates our relationships to be healthy and whole. He wants us divided against each other. Sometimes we forget the real enemy is not our brother or sister in Christ. Rather it is the devil, who wants us to believe our prayers are not effective, or that only the elite can pray and have results. But Scripture teaches us that we all have a part in sharing one another's burdens and praying for God's healing hand to touch others. God uses you in different ways, with different gifts—that's why community is so powerful.

THE ANOINTING

The first way God might use you in healing is with the help of the anointing. The Word tells us God anointed Jesus of Nazareth with the Holy Spirit and with power. After that anointing, Jesus went about doing good and healing everyone who was oppressed of the devil because God was with Him (see Acts 10:38). I looked up the word oppressed and found that it means "to dominate or exercise lordship." When Jesus healed people, He exercised His authority over Satan's domination.

Scripture says that the anointing breaks the yoke. Jesus was able to heal because He was anointed with the Holy Spirit. It was the presence of God Who performed the healing work.

When you are sick, you are being oppressed or dominated by illness; the Word says all those whom Jesus healed were oppressed of the devil. The anointing breaks the yoke, or the bondage. Jesus has the power to heal anyone. When He was resurrected, He left us to do even greater works. Christ is the "Anointed One", and we are His ambassadors; He equipped us with the gifts of the Spirit. First John 2:20 and 27 says:

"But you have an anointing from the Holy One, and all of you know the truth. ... As for you, the anointing you received from him remains in you, and you do not need anyone to teach you. But as his anointing teaches you about all things and as that anointing is real, not counterfeit—just as it has taught you, remain in him (NIV)."

I heard a young pastor and theologian tell how God had transformed his mind and heart about healing. He was a cessationist—meaning, all miracles have ceased since the Apostles. He accepted an invitation to speak at a meeting in a church, thinking the pastor was of the same mind and opinion. But he soon found himself to be a captive audience. At this meeting, he saw the healing power of Jesus on an anointed man break the bondage of sickness. Today this pastor is telling everyone who will listen that Jesus is healing bodies today. The anointing is the presence of God and His power, which is available to us today.

WORDS OF HEALING
TEXT: 1 Corinthians 12:14-31 (NIV)

The Body of Christ and the Gifts of the Spirit

14 Now the body is not made up of one part but of many. 15 If the foot should say, "Because I am not a hand, I do not belong to the body," it would not for that reason cease to be part of the body. 16 And if the ear should say, "Because I am not an eye, I do not belong to the body," it would not for that reason cease to be part of the body. 17 If the whole body were an eye, where would the sense of hearing be? If the whole body were an ear, where would the sense of smell be? 18 But in fact God has arranged the parts in the body, every one of them, just as he wanted them to be. 19 If they were all one part, where would the body be? 20 As it is, there are many parts, but one body. 21 The eye cannot say to the hand, "I don't need you!" And the head cannot say to the feet, "I don't need you!" 22 On the contrary, those parts of the body that seem to be weaker are indispensable, 23 and the parts that we think are less honorable we treat with special honor. And the parts that are unpresentable are treated with special modesty, 24 while our presentable parts need no special treatment. But God has combined the members of the body and has given greater honor to the parts that lacked it, 25 so that there should be no division in the body, but that its parts should have equal concern for each other. 26 If one part suffers, every part suffers with it; if one part is honored, every part rejoices with it.

27 Now you are the body of Christ, and each one of you is a part of it. 28 And in the church God has appointed first of all apostles, second prophets, third teachers, then workers of miracles, also those having gifts of healing, those able to help others, those with gifts of administration, and those speaking in different kinds of tongues. 29 Are all apostles? Are all prophets? Are all teachers? Do all work miracles? 30 Do all have gifts of healing? Do all speak in tongues? Do all interpret? 31 But eagerly desire the greater gifts. And now I will show you the most excellent way."

    Here we see in verse 30 that some are even given the gift of healing. All these gifts are possible through the power of the Holy Spirit, and these were given to us as a gift, yet the Body has not taken advantage of what God has generously given to His church.

    Some of you may have taken a spiritual gifts test and I think they can be helpful; but, we also have to be mindful that the Spirit moves as He wills. As such, He can anoint any of us with one of these gifts for a situation to accomplish His will. Many times, we do tend to walk consistently in a certain gift, but the Spirit can give any of us the anointing or the gift of healing. Paul also wants us to keep this in check. Love is supreme and we must work together.

    Jesus healed with love and compassion (ironically, the next chapter in Corinthians is known as the "Love Chapter"—1 Corinthians 13). The awareness of God's love is the foundation of everything I can believe or receive. Everything God has done for us comes out of His great love.

    "And Jesus went forth, and saw a great multitude, and was moved with compassion toward them, and he healed their sick" (Matthew 14:14, KJV).

INSIGHTS ON HEALING

1. From the list of gifts or charisms listed in the 1 Corinthians 12 passage, which ones have you experienced personally?

2. Why do you think the gifts have been such a divisive issue in our churches?

3. Name some of the barriers that can quench the Spirit when we gather together to pray for healing.

HEALING ENCOUNTER

What I love about gathering people together for teaching on healing is that it allows for an atmosphere where corporate faith can dwell. As you go through this study, you will have the opportunity to hear the faith of others, and you will have prayed for people you would perhaps have never prayed for. The more we come together, the more we bring our faith together, the quicker healing will happen and the more dramatic it will be.

Sometimes you think a certain person is spiritual, but you really don't know. You don't know where their faith is. Get them to pray anyway, right? That is very important. So as you lead a study or participate, don't write anyone off—but invite even those you think may not come. Let God open up hearts toward each other. I believe when we gather like that, the anointing for healing does come.

I know the times I've felt most anointed to teach was when I had the faith of others behind me. One recent service I led, I asked everyone and their dog to pray. I really had this request way out there, to please pray for me because I was going to preach on this whole topic of healing. People were calling me to let me know I was being lifted up, texting me, leaving messages. I was very encouraged by their personal touches alone. But then the meeting started and I felt the anointing so strongly. I knew exactly why; it was the corporate faith of others.

We need this—we need each other. The enemy continues to try and divide His church, His people, so that we can't join our faith with other believers. I believe the anointing comes and the gifts manifest themselves naturally when we are united. So keep gathering together!

HEALING ACTION POINT

You may be going through this study alone or with a group. Whatever your circumstances, pick one person you've been praying for out of your prayer journal. Ask your group to pray, those outside your group, anyone who might be willing to pray for this specific request. Make it a point to bring the faith of others together and see what God does. Record any answers to prayer and reflect on how you may have personally experienced His anointing.

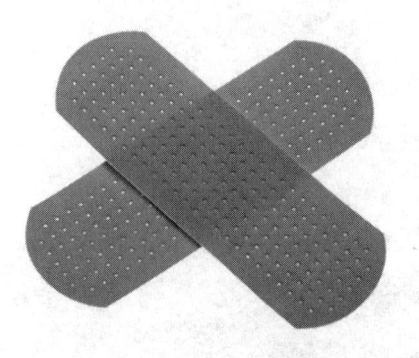

Notes:

CHAPTER THIRTEEN

METHODS GOD USES

"God did extraordinary miracles through Paul, so that even handkerchiefs and aprons that had touched him were taken to the sick, and their illnesses were cured and the evil spirits left them" (Acts 19:11-12, NIV).

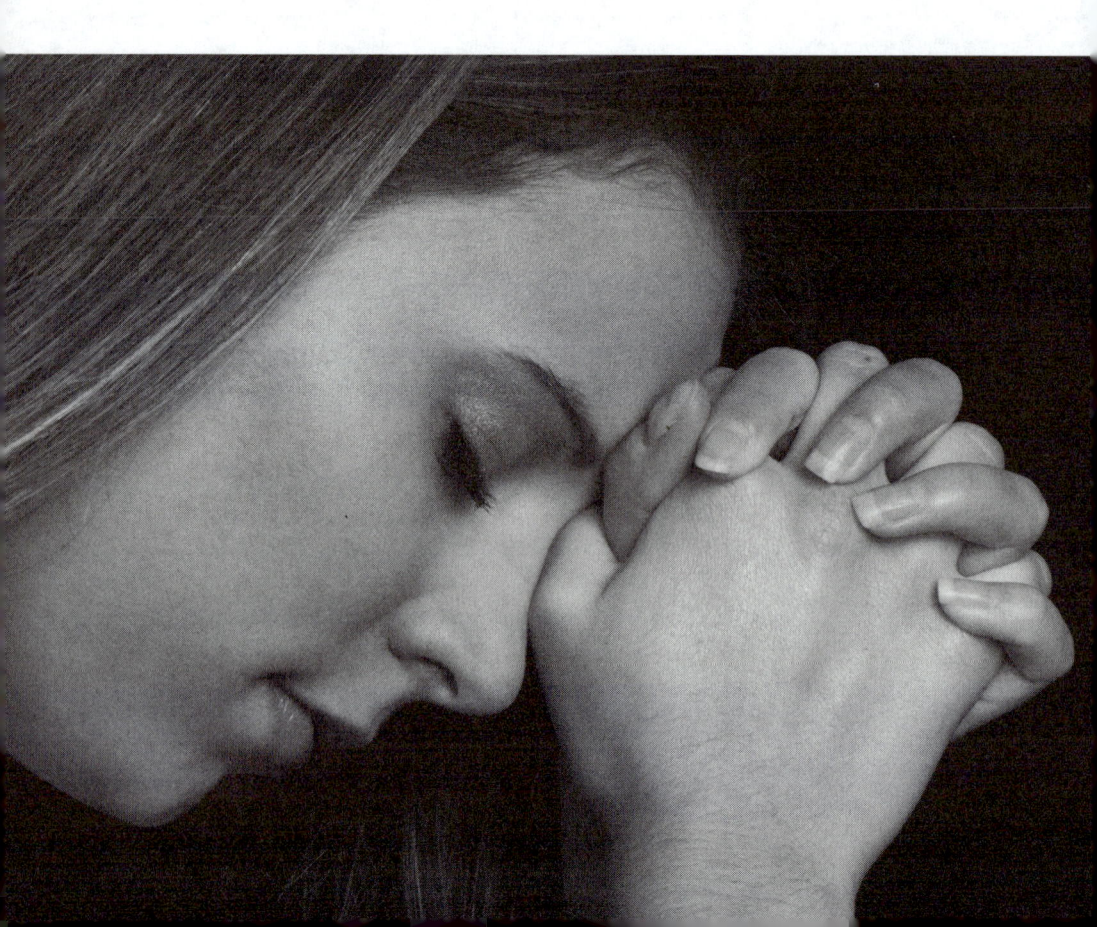

God is so intent on healing us and making us whole that He has a myriad of ways to do it. I've actually found seventeen different ways in which God heals. He knows we are such diverse people and that we all respond differently in different situations. We are all varied in our personalities, our backgrounds, and our experiences. God is gracious to meet us wherever we are. And God certainly isn't limited to any method in the healing process.

Sometimes God uses a point of contact, like a prayer cloth. Maybe you think of this as the "Pentecostal way." This is biblical and we have Scripture where we know people were healed from a physical item:

"God did extraordinary miracles through Paul, so that even handkerchiefs and aprons that had touched him were taken to the sick, and their illnesses were cured and the evil spirits left them" (Acts 19:11-12).

Other times God uses the power of His spoken Word and healing happens in miraculous ways. Psalm 107:20 says, *"He sent his word, and healed them, and delivered them from their destructions."* Sometimes it is just that simple. There are examples in the Bible where Jesus didn't go visit the sick; rather, He spoke the Word of healing and the individual was made well. Once when Jesus was teaching in Cana, a nobleman from Capernaum came to Jesus and begged Him to go and heal his son who was at the point of death. This situation was critical; time was of the essence. Instead of going to Capernaum, Jesus said, "Go thy way; thy son liveth." The father believed Jesus, went home, and found his son well—healed at the very moment Jesus sent His Word to him.

One big method that all of us can do very comfortably is using prayer. We don't have to be in a healing service, we don't have to have hands laid on us, and we don't have to be anointed with oil. Simply put, God answers prayer. James 5:15 tells us, *"And the prayer of faith shall save the sick..."*

Another way the LORD ministers healing is through a "word of knowledge." Some of you may not be familiar with this gift, but it is mentioned in 1 Corinthians 12:8. I have found the LORD uses this a lot with me in my teaching meetings. He'll often give me a "word of knowledge" about the physical needs of many in the congregation. It isn't something you had previous knowledge about, but it is when the LORD graces you with His knowledge.

Prayer and fasting is probably the method that takes the most discipline from us. The body is seldom comfortable when it is deprived of food. Setting aside time to pray when you could be eating takes determination. Nevertheless, the rewards are great. Jesus cast a demon out of a child and said, "This kind goeth not out but by prayer and fasting."

There are other ways we see in Scripture as well, and all of these methods can be used effectively when we come together corporately. My prayer for you as we end our study is that you'd be open to being used in whatever method God is calling you to move in.

WORDS OF HEALING
TEXT: 2 Kings 5:1-19 (NIV)

Naaman Healed of Leprosy

₁Now Naaman was commander of the army of the king of Aram. He was a great man in the sight of his master and highly regarded, because through him the LORD had given victory to Aram. He was a valiant soldier, but he had leprosy. ₂Now bands from Aram had gone out and had taken captive a young girl from Israel, and she served Naaman's wife. ₃She said to her mistress, "If only my master would see the prophet who is in Samaria! He would cure him of his leprosy."
₄Naaman went to his master and told him what the girl from Israel had said. ₅"By all means, go," the king of Aram replied. "I will send a letter to the king of Israel." So Naaman left, taking with him ten talents of silver, six thousand shekels of gold and ten sets of clothing. ₆The letter that he took to the king of Israel read: "With this letter I am sending my servant Naaman to you so that you may cure him of his leprosy."
₇As soon as the king of Israel read the letter, he tore his robes and said, "Am I God? Can I kill and bring back to life? Why does this fellow send someone to me to be cured of his leprosy? See how he is trying to pick a quarrel with me!"
₈When Elisha the man of God heard that the king of Israel had torn his robes, he sent him this message: "Why have you torn your robes? Have the man come to me and he will know that there is a prophet in Israel." ₉So Naaman went with his horses and chariots and stopped at the door of Elisha's house. ₁₀Elisha sent a messenger to say to him, "Go, wash yourself seven times in the Jordan, and your flesh will be restored and you will be cleansed."
₁₁But Naaman went away angry and said, "I thought that he would surely come out to me and stand and call on the name of the LORD his God, wave his hand over the spot and cure me of my leprosy. ₁₂Are not Abana and Pharpar, the rivers of Damascus, better than any of the waters of Israel? Couldn't I wash in them and be cleansed?" So he turned and went off in a rage.
₁₃Naaman's servants went to him and said, "My father, if the prophet had told you to do some great thing, would you not have done it? How much more, then, when he tells you, 'Wash and be cleansed'!" ₁₄So he went down and dipped himself in the Jordan seven times, as the man of God had told him, and his flesh was restored and became clean like that of a young boy.
₁₅Then Naaman and all his attendants went back to the man of God. He stood before him and said, "Now I know that there is no God in all the world except in Israel. Please accept now a gift from your servant."
₁₆The prophet answered, "As surely as the LORD lives, whom I serve, I will not accept a thing." And even though Naaman urged him, he refused.
₁₇"If you will not," said Naaman, "please let me, your servant, be given as much earth as a pair of mules can carry, for your servant will never again make burnt offerings and sacrifices to any other god but the LORD. ₁₈But may the LORD forgive your servant for this one thing: When my master enters the temple of Rimmon to bow down and he is leaning on my arm and I bow there also—when I bow down in the temple of Rimmon, may the LORD forgive your servant for this."
₁₉"Go in peace," Elisha said.

INSIGHTS ON HEALING

1. What method of healing did Elisha use to bring about healing to Naaman?

2. It's important to remember that the method itself is never magical, nor is it ever the source of power. What are some ways we can focus on God's power, no matter what method is used?

3. Which method discussed in this chapter are you most comfortable with? Uncomfortable? Note which one you would like to learn more about.

HEALING ENCOUNTER

I'm personally so grateful to know God has the right method for every situation. I remember the first time I took hold of sending out the Word to someone; it was when my mother was told she had a brain tumor. We were out of town when I received the news that x-rays indicated there was a growth. Fear tried to grip my mind; my mother was alone, and we weren't there to pray for her. I was desperate; I felt I had to do something. Then the Holy Spirit brought to mind, "He sent His Word and healed them."

Immediately I formed a mental picture of that Word, like an arrow, piercing my mother's brain. Then I saw the arrow strike a dark spot, and the thing just exploded. I called my mother when Wally and I returned home, and I asked her to go to the doctor for another x-ray. The x-ray came back with no sign of a tumor on my mother's brain. Glory to God! His Word never wears out or loses its power!

I hope you have been encouraged by this study and realize in a fresh way how God wants to use you to lift up others and be apart of His healing ministry.

HEALING ACTION POINT

Refer to Appendix D, Healing Miracles of Jesus Guide. Take time to reflect on all the ways in which Jesus healed people. Gather in groups of three or more and begin praying for your own healing and the healing of others. See how each individual is led in light of the methods we've looked at together in this chapter. After your time of prayer, turn to the back to your prayer journal and note what you experienced.

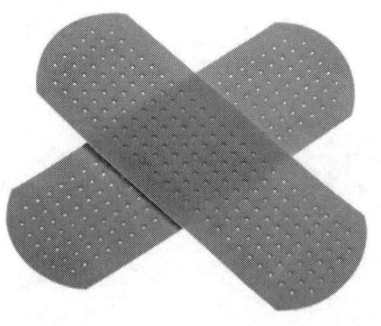

Notes:

section 5

APPENDICES

APPENDIX A: HEALING PRAYERS/JOURNAL

A prayer journal has been provided for you as you go through this study. As you interact with the material, meditate on scriptures, and pray with others, log your reflections. It's important to take time and praise God for the answers to prayer. I'm confident you will have much to give praise about. –Marilyn

Date: _____

Prayer Request:

_____
_____
_____
_____
_____
_____
_____
_____
_____
_____
_____

Scriptures You are Praying Over Others:

_____
_____
_____
_____
_____
_____
_____
_____
_____

Prayers of Healing Answered:

_____
_____
_____
_____
_____
_____
_____

Date: _____

Prayer Request:

_____
_____
_____
_____
_____
_____
_____
_____
_____
_____

Scriptures You are Praying Over Others:

_____
_____
_____
_____
_____
_____
_____
_____
_____

Prayers of Healing Answered:

_____
_____
_____
_____
_____
_____
_____

Date: _____

Prayer Request:
_____
_____
_____
_____
_____
_____
_____
_____
_____
_____
_____

Scriptures You are Praying Over Others:
_____
_____
_____
_____
_____
_____
_____
_____
_____

Prayers of Healing Answered:
_____
_____
_____
_____
_____
_____
_____

Date: _____

Prayer Request:

_____
_____
_____
_____
_____
_____
_____
_____
_____
_____

Scriptures You are Praying Over Others:

_____
_____
_____
_____
_____
_____
_____
_____
_____

Prayers of Healing Answered:

_____
_____
_____
_____
_____
_____

Date: _____

Prayer Request:
_____
_____
_____
_____
_____
_____
_____
_____
_____
_____

Scriptures You are Praying Over Others:
_____
_____
_____
_____
_____
_____
_____
_____
_____

Prayers of Healing Answered:
_____
_____
_____
_____
_____
_____
_____

Date: _____

Prayer Request:
_____
_____
_____
_____
_____
_____
_____
_____
_____

Scriptures You are Praying Over Others:
_____
_____
_____
_____
_____
_____
_____
_____

Prayers of Healing Answered:
_____
_____
_____
_____
_____
_____
_____

Date: _____

Prayer Request:

_____
_____
_____
_____
_____
_____
_____
_____
_____
_____
_____

Scriptures You are Praying Over Others:

_____
_____
_____
_____
_____
_____
_____
_____
_____

Prayers of Healing Answered:

_____
_____
_____
_____
_____
_____
_____

Date: _____

Prayer Request:

_____
_____
_____
_____
_____
_____
_____
_____
_____
_____

Scriptures You are Praying Over Others:

_____
_____
_____
_____
_____
_____
_____
_____
_____
_____

Prayers of Healing Answered:

_____
_____
_____
_____
_____
_____
_____

Date: _____

Prayer Request:

_____
_____
_____
_____
_____
_____
_____
_____
_____
_____

Scriptures You are Praying Over Others:

_____
_____
_____
_____
_____
_____
_____
_____
_____

Prayers of Healing Answered:

_____
_____
_____
_____
_____
_____
_____

Date: _____

Prayer Request:
_____
_____
_____
_____
_____
_____
_____
_____
_____

Scriptures You are Praying Over Others:
_____
_____
_____
_____
_____
_____
_____
_____

Prayers of Healing Answered:
_____
_____
_____
_____
_____
_____
_____

Date: _____

Prayer Request:
_____
_____
_____
_____
_____
_____
_____
_____
_____
_____
_____

Scriptures You are Praying Over Others:
_____
_____
_____
_____
_____
_____
_____
_____

Prayers of Healing Answered:
_____
_____
_____
_____
_____
_____
_____

APPENDIX B: SPEAK THE WORD

Speak The Word
Marilyn Hickey
Marilyn Hickey Ministries
PO Box 6598
Englewood, CO 80155-6598
Unless otherwise indicated,
all Scripture quotations are taken from
the King James Version of the Bible
ISBN 1-56441-166-4
Revised 1983 Edition
Printed in the United States of America
Copyright © 1982 by Marilyn Hickey
All Rights Reserved

SPEAK THE WORD

Your tongue is the most powerful weapon and force of your life. Proverbs states that the tongue has the power of life and death in it. In James 3, James states that you can control your whole body by the small member you have, called the tongue. As a rudder guides a ship and a bit in the horse's mouth causes him to go the right direction, so also your tongue can guide your thoughts, your emotions, and your body in paths of prosperity and success and be a tremendous power for good.
But on the negative side, your tongue can be used to damage and destroy your physical body, your thought life, and your emotional reactions. Corrupt words can destroy those about is, for the Psalmist states that words are like the piercing of swords. You set on fire the course of nature by what you speak because hell acts on your words. Eve had to speak wrong words before Satan could act. Hell can act only on your words, so every negative word you speak sets hell into activity. This is why God spoke to Joshua (Joshua 1:8) said,

> "This book of the law shall not depart from your mouth, but you
> shall meditate on it day and night, so that you may be careful to
> do according to all that is written in it: for then you will have success (NASV)."

This little verse in Joshua is the key to all prosperity and success. In fact, this is the Only place the word success is found in the Bible. Speaking God's Word can make you successful in every area of your life.

What about words spoken against us and our loved ones? Will those negative confessions set hell into activity in our lives? As always God's Word has an answer. It is found in Isaiah 54:17, "No weapon that is formed against thee shall prosper and every tongue that shall rise against thee is judgment thou shalt condemn. This is the heritage of the servants of the Lord and their righteousness is of me." Condemn wrong words spoken against you and ours in the name of Jesus. Never condemn the person who speaks, only the words spoken against you. Then these negative word weapons cannot harm you.

Defeat the enemy today. Speak the following words of Life every day. In harassing times, speak them three times a day. God's Word works. Try it—you'll love it! Speaking aloud causes your spirit man to hear. This is the way to grow strong in spirit. Make your faith effective. Say the Word, say the Word, say the Word. "Let the words of my mouth be acceptable in your sight today, O Lord."

I have an anointing from the Holy One, and today Jesus is made unto me wisdom, righteousness, sanctification and redemption, for I have the mind of Christ. Through wisdom I build my house and by understanding it is established (1 John 2:20; 1 Corinthians 1:30; 1 Corinthians 2:16; James 3:17; Proverbs 24:3).

God's wisdom will put me over today for God's wisdom is from above. As I speak His words of wisdom. I will bring peace and mercy to my situation. I shall not walk in darkness today for the Holy Spirit will guide me into all truth. The Lord will give me understanding in all things and wisdom and knowledge shall stabilize my times for I have the mind of Christ (James 3:17; John 16:13; 1 Corinthians 1:30; 2 Timothy 2:7; Isaiah 33:6; 1 Corinthians 2:16).

Satan cannot overcome me for God has given me a mouth and wisdom the enemy cannot gainsay or resist (Luke 21:15).

I walk not in darkness for it is given unto me to know the mysteries of the kingdom. The Lord instructs me and teaches me in the way that I should go: He guides me with His eye (Matthew 13:11; Romans 1:19; Psalm 32:8).

Today I am persuaded that I am filled with goodness, all knowledge, and ability to help my brother. I am good in the sight of God and He gives me wisdom, and knowledge, and joy (Romans 15:14; Ecclesiastes 2:26).

I am filled with the knowledge of the Lord's will in all wisdom and spiritual understanding; I am a new creation in Christ; I am His workmanship created in Christ Jesus. Because of this, I have His wisdom and my decisions are ordered of Him (Colossians 1:9; 2 Corinthians 5:17; 1 Corinthians 2:16),

God, the father of my Lord Jesus Christ gives unto me the spirit of wisdom and revelation and my eyes are enlightened that I may know the hope of the glory of His inheritance in me and the exceeding greatness of His power that flows through me (Ephesians 1:17-19).

JOY

Today I shall have joy because I shall speak words that bring life to me and others. The joy of the Lord is the strength of my life, so I can do all things through Christ who strengthens me (Proverbs 15:23; Proverbs 25:11; Nehemiah 8:10; Philippians 4:13).

No corrupt communication shall come out of my mouth today for I speak words of faith and edification. Therefore, my words bring life and joy (Ephesians 4:29).

I will have joy by the answers of my mouth so today I speak His words of power. I will enter into the joy of the Lord today and I will be a helper of the joy of others. I will speak words of faith to others (Proverbs 15:23: Matthew 25:23; 2 Corinthians 1:24).

I love righteousness and hate iniquity; therefore God, even my God, has anointed me with the oil of gladness above my fellows. I put my trust in the Lord and rejoice; I shout for joy because He defends me :I love His name and am joyful in Him (Hebrews 1:9; Psalm 5:11).

My heart rejoices in Him because I trust in His holy name. I greatly rejoice in the Lord, my soul is joyful in my God; for He has clothed me with the garments of salvation. He has covered me with the robe of righteousness. Your Word is unto me the joy and rejoicing of my heart, for I am called by your name. O Lord God of Hosts (Isaiah 61:10; Jeremiah 15:16).

HEALTH AND WEALTH

The Lord sent His Word and healed me and delivered me from all destruction. I serve the Lord and He blesses my food and drink; and He takes away sickness from me and my family; He heals all our diseases (Psalm 107:20; Exodus 23:25; Psalm 103:3b).

The Spirit of Him that raised Jesus from the dead dwells in me; therefore He that raised up Christ from the dead has quickened my mortal body, making it immune to every sickness and disease (Romans 8:11).

All my needs are met in Christ Jesus for my God supplies all my needs according to His riches in glory. Christ has redeemed me from the curse of poverty, sickness and spiritual death; and because I am the seed of Abraham, blessing He will bless me and multiplying He will multiply me. I receive the bountifulness (Philippians 4:19; Galatians 3:13; Hebrews 6:14).
I give and it is given unto me, good measure, pressed down, shaken together and running over (Luke 6:38).
Today I rejoice in all that I put my hand to. He blesses the labor of my hands. I am happy and all is well with me and my household needs are met abundantly through Him who supplies all my needs (Psalm 128:1-2; Deuteronomy 12:7, 18b).
Wealth and riches shall be in my house and my righteousness endures forever (Psalm 112:3).

SAFETY AND RELEASE FROM FEAR
Today there is safety for me and my loved ones for there is no wisdom nor understanding nor counsel against the Lord (Proverbs 21:30).

I hear the voice of the Lord through His Word. Therefore, I dwell safely and am quiet from fear of evil (Proverbs 1:33).
My loved ones and I are delivered from the powers of darkness and translated into the Kingdom of His dear Son. No evil shall befall, neither shall any plague come near my dwelling. I overcome all the fiery darts of the enemy and nothing can harm me because greater is He that is in me that he that is in the world (Colossians 1:13; Psalm 91:10; Ephesians 6:16; 1 John 4:4).

I am established in righteousness: I am far from oppression; for I do not fear; and from terror; for it shall not come near me. God has not given me the spirit of fear, but of power, and of love, and of a sound mind (Isaiah 54:14; 2 Timothy 1:7).

The Lord is my refuge and my fortress; my God; in Him will I trust. He has given me power to tread on serpents and scorpions, and over all the power of the enemy; so nothing shall by any means hurt me (Psalm 91:2; Luke 10:19).

FAMILY
God has set before me life and death, blessing and cursing: therefore I choose life; that both my seed and I may live. I know that my home shall be in peace; and I shall visit my habitation and shall not sin. I know also that my seed shall be great, and my offspring as the grass of the earth. The wicked are overthrown, and are not; but my house shall stand (Deuteronomy 30:19; Job 5:24-25; Proverbs 12:7).

I believe on the Lord Jesus Christ, and I am saved, and my house (Acts 16:31).

The seed of the righteous shall be delivered. The Lord is righteousness: he has cut asunder all the cords of the wicked in my household (Proverbs 11:21; Psalm 129:4).

My children are wise and make my heart glad: they are taught of the Lord and great is the peace of my children (Proverbs 27:11; Isaiah 54:13).

I train up my child in the way he should go; and when he is old, he will not depart from it (Proverbs 22:6).

I teach God's Word to my children, speaking of it when I sit in my house, and when I walk by the way, when I lie down, and when I rise up. I tell my children of it, and my children tell their children and their children another generation (Deuteronomy 11:19; Joel 1:3).

My sons and daughters (name them) will not forget God's teachings but will let their hearts keep His commandments. For length of days and years of life and peace will they add to them. They do not let kindness and truth leave them; but bind them about their necks and write them upon the tablets of their hearts. So will they find favor and good repute in the sight of God and man (Proverbs 3:1-4).

You, God, will not allow my children's feet to slip or to be moved except toward you. You keep them and will not slumber (Psalm 121:3).

Lord, you are righteous; you have cut asunder the thick cords (lists specific sins) by which the wicked Satan enslaved us (Psalm 129:4).

UNCONDITIONAL LOVE
I let love be without dissimulation. I abhor that which is evil, and I cleave to that which is good (Romans 12:9).

And this I pray, that my love abounds yet more and more in knowledge and in all judgment; and I know the love of Christ, which passes knowledge, and I am filled with all the fullness of God (Philippians 1:9; Ephesians 3:19).

RELATIONSHIPS
I thank you, Father, that you surround me with favor as with a shield and therefore, I have favor with my family and co-workers and also with all the people with whom I come in contact today (Psalm 5:12).

Father, I thank you that, because we are both reconciled to Jesus by the blood of His cross, _____ and I are also reconciled to each other, regardless of anything we have done to each other I the past (Colossians 1:20-21).

FOR THOSE IN AUTHORITY

Today I pray for my President and those in authority over me that their hearts are in the hand of the Lord and He turns them whithersoever He will (Proverbs 21:1).

Our nation, pastors and church are blessed because our God is the Lord and we are the people He has chosen for His inheritance (Psalm 33:12).

The body of Christ and I are the righteousness of God; therefore I exalt this nation and bind principalities, powers, rulers of darkness and spiritual wickedness and render them ineffective against my nation, my church, my family, and myself, in the Name of Jesus (2 Corinthians 5:12; Proverbs 14:34; Ephesians 6:12).

Notes:

APPENDIX C: THE HEALING POWER OF COMMUNION

Communion Service

Take time during this group study to plan communion together. You don't need special bread or juice, just whatever you can bring together. There are various ways to take it together, so have someone in your group plan the method and how you will join one another in this meal of celebration. All that is required is that you believe in Jesus Christ as your Lord and Savior. I do believe it is a time when people are healed in miraculous ways and when the Holy Spirit is at work.
Communion is something Jesus asked us to do often, to remember His sacrifice and the forgiveness and healing that is available to us. Communion is union with Him. Remembering what is already done and bringing it into present tense. It's a time to celebrate what He has already done for us. We don't have to work to get it; we celebrate it.
I believe taking the bread and the juice together opens us up to a special grace of God. It's an intimate time when I ask from Jesus what I really need. It really is about what He can do miraculously inside of me as I remember His body, broken for me.

Paul had a great understanding of communion. By the spirit He received it. Get in the Holy Spirit, like Paul. What God has provided for you, receive this by the Lord Jesus. Paul wasn't there in the Upper Room when Jesus served the disciples but He knew by the Spirit; He knew what went on. The same presence that was with Paul is the same for you today.

Communion reminds us of our connection as family, our relationships. I just need Jesus to be with me. That is one reason why we take communion, and it is a time to invite his presence to be with us. It's a time set apart for us to engage in Him, not just traditional going through the motions, but where we invite His presence.

1 Corinthians 11:24: the first thing Jesus did before breaking the bread with His disciples was to give thanks to His Father. When we rush in to the presence, and we forget to be grateful, we miss a blessing. We need to put our requests on hold for a bit. Jesus was giving thanks for the fact his body was going to be broken. I believe thanks give you strength. We often want the blessing before giving thanks. Jesus did it in faith.

"Take eat this is my body. Do this in remembrance of me." The purpose of it is to be healed. To be whole. Remember what I've done: By His stripes we are healed. Jesus came to reconcile us from our sins.

Suggested Elements of a Communion Service:
Praise and Thanksgiving
Confession
Acknowledge your needs
Take the Elements together
End in prayer and thanks

SCRIPTURE SUGGESTIONS TO READ CORPORATELY:

1 Corinthians 11:27-29

1 John 1:9

Ruth 2:4

1 Samuel 17:37

Lamentations 3:41

Isaiah 6:3

Matthew 21:9, Mark 11:9-10, John 12:13

Hebrews 4:15

1 John 2:2

1 Corinthians 11:25-26

John 6:53-59

Acts 17:28

1 Corinthians 5:7-8a

John 6:56

Genesis 9:4

Record in your prayer journals your reflections, what the Spirit speaks to you, your group, and any healings that take place during the service you planned.

Notes:

APPENDIX D: HEALING MIRACLES OF JESUS

The Healing Miracles of Jesus

There are so many powerful scriptures of healing we can pray for one another. I've listed a quick reference guide for you if you are searching for one that speaks to the need of another. As a faith building exercise, I encourage you to read about the healing miracles of Jesus.

Jesus drives out an evil spirit in Capernaum: Mark 1:21-28; Luke 4:36-37

The healing of Simon's mother-in-law: Matthew 8:14-15; Mark 1:29-31; Luke 4:38-39

Healings during evening time: Matthew 8:16-17; Mark 1:32-34; Luke 4:40-41

The leper: Matthew 8:1-4; Mark 1:40-44; Luke 5:12-16

The paralytic: Matthew 9:1-8; Mark 2:1-12; Luke 5:17-26

The withered hand: Matthew 12:9-14; Mark 3:1-6; Luke 6:6-11

Healing in Galilee: Matthew 12:15-21; Mark 3:7-12; Luke 6:17-19

The demoniacs of Garasene: Matthew 8:28-34; Mark 5:1-20; Luke 8:26-39

Jairus' daughter and the woman with the issue of blood: Matthew 9:18-26; Mark 5:21-23; Luke 8:40-56

Healing at Gennesaret: Matthew 14:34-3; Mark 6:53-56

The Syrophenician (Canaanite woman) Matthew 15:21-28; Mark 7:24-30

The deaf mute: Mark 7:31-37

Blind man at Bethsaida: Mark 8:22-26

The epileptic boy: Matthew 17:14-21; mark 9:14-29; Luke 9:37-43

Blind Bartimaeus: Matthew 20:29-34; Mark 10:46-52; Luke 18:35-43

The centurion's servant: Matthew 8:5-13; Luke 7:1-10

Healing Miracles of Jesus

Healings in the Galilean synagogues: Matthew 4:23

The two blind men: Matthew 9:27-31

The dumb demoniac: Matthew 9:32-34

Healings throughout Galilee: Matthew 9:35

The blind/dumb demoniac: Matthew 12:22

Healings in the wilderness: Matthew 14:14

Healings on the mountain: Matthew 15: 29-31

Healings near the Jordan: Matthew 19:2

Healings in the temple: Matthew 21:14

Widow's son at Nain: Luke 7:11-17

Healings to prove Messiahship to John: Luke 7:21

Healings at Bethsaida: Luke 9:11

The crippled woman: Luke 13:10-13

The man with dropsy: Luke 14:1-6

The ear of the high priests' servant: Luke 22:51

Signs in Jerusalem: John 2:23-25

The official's son: John 4:46-54

The lame man at Bethesda: John 5:1-15

The man born blind: John 9:1-34

The raising of Lazarus from the dead: John 11:1-44

Notes:

Notes:

Notes:

Notes: